DEATH IN THE POT

MORTON SATIN

THE IMPACT OF FOOD POISONING ON HISTORY

DEATH IN THE POT

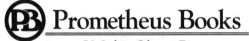 **Prometheus Books**
59 John Glenn Drive
Amherst, New York 14228–2197

Published 2007 by Prometheus Books

Inquiries should be addressed to
Prometheus Books
59 John Glenn Drive
Amherst, New York 14228–2197
VOICE: 716–691–0133, ext. 210
FAX: 716–691–0137
WWW.PROMETHEUSBOOKS.COM

11 10 09 08 07   5 4 3 2 1

Library of Congress Cataloging-in-Publication Data

Satin, Morton.
    Death in the pot : the impact of food poisoning on history / Morton Satin.
        p. cm.
    Includes bibliographical references and index.
    ISBN 978–1–59102–514–6
    1. Food poisoning—History. 2. Food contamination—History. 3. Diseases and history. I. Title. [DNLM: 1. Food Poisoning—History. 2. Food Contamination. WC 11.1 S253d 2007]

RC143.S28 2007
614.5—dc22

                                                                    2007022201

Printed in the United States of America on acid-free paper

For Jerry

CONTENTS

PART IV. THE MODERN ERA

ACKNOWLEDGMENTS

I would like to thank Mr. Ed Knappman of New England Publishing Associates for suggesting this book and providing encouragement and guidance throughout its preparation. I would also like to thank Suzanne Junod and John Swann of the FDA Library for their patience and assistance in reviewing historical records related to the Ginger Jake episode. I am particularly grateful to Linda Greenspan Regan of Prometheus Books for keeping me on track and for her efforts in turning the manuscript into a finished product. Finally, I would like to thank my wife, Miriam, for her patience and support through the course of this book.

FOREWORD

Coming from an educational background in microbiology and a lifetime of working experience in the food industry, I naturally have a strong personal and professional interest in the subject of food poisoning. During the course of my career, I always relied on the preponderance of scientific data to make my decisions and to inform consumers on complex matters of health and safety related to food.

When Ed Knappman of New England Publishing Associates first suggested a book on the history of food poisoning, I was caught in a dilemma. One of the great difficulties in writing a book on the history of food poisoning is that there is very limited scientific material to go by. Our understanding of spoilage and disease is not much more than a century old. Having been trained to arrive at conclusions only after evaluating strong scientific evidence, how would it be possible to state with any degree of credibility which events in history could have resulted from food poisoning?

Despite that problem, the subject was just too interesting to drop, and I started looking into some of the historical records related to food poisoning in the past. While there was no scientific evidence of the agents or microorganisms that may have caused several unlikely events, in many cases the descriptions of the diseases themselves were so detailed that it was possible to infer what caused the outbreaks.

More research revealed that disease outbreaks were linked to a great many major events in history. Suddenly, the bizarre behavior of some of civilization's great leaders could be explained. Epic biblical events could be plausibly explained in scientific terms. It was possible to rationally speculate that tiny molecules or microorganisms had as crucial an influence on the flow of human events as did great ideas and principles. It wasn't long before I was hooked on the subject.

Poisoning, through food, beverages, or other means, has always had a particular fascination for us because of its association with crime and romance. However, we seldom consider food poisoning as an agent of social or economic change. Yet, silent and unseen, agents of food poisoning have had a tremendous impact on the course of history and continue to do so today.

This book makes no pretense of uncovering masses of new original research but puts together information from a variety of published work. The goal of this compilation is to demonstrate that some of history's greatest events were controlled by nature's tiniest elements.

Morton Satin
Rockville, Maryland
October 28, 2006

PREFACE
SILESIA
Autumn of 12,800 BC

Hooded, the figure moved swiftly and silently through the dark woods. After hearing the distant summons of the great horn, he quickly and carefully damped the embers of his fire and proceeded warily into the night. The thin crescent of moon cast a dim, feathery light on the soft forest floor, allowing him to easily make out the details of the thick underbrush. Despite the thickness of his rough leather footwear, his feet delicately sensed everything on the ground beneath him. The distance between his secluded cavern and the overhung limestone cliffs that sheltered the tribe's permanent settlement was not great. The heavy night air easily carried the sounds of animals getting ready to hunt or arguing among themselves. The tone and intensity of the nighttime insect cacophony served as his weather barometer, letting him know what the coming hours or days would bring. The Shaman traveled the forest with confidence and purpose. He had no fear of the creatures of the night because he was one of them, and they knew him to be so.

The signs of another winter were beginning to appear. Even though they were still green, the leaves were getting thinner and tasted drier between his cracked lips; soon they would change color and drift to the ground. The air was beginning to feel moister between his fingers and heavier when he exhaled into his cupped hand. The penetrating scents and challenging calls of the animals getting ready for the mating season were becoming much more obvious. The rhythms were unchanged throughout his life. This was going to be the forty-sixth winter that he could remember, which made him an old man—the oldest member of the tribe, by far.

The Shaman lived his life at a spiritual and physical distance from the rest of the tribe. Dressed in the head and skins of the great bear, he would visit them during the time of the full moon to guide them in worshiping the gods of the hunt, but other than that, he had very little contact with them. Of course, the tribe members could always summon him with the great horn whenever the need arose, but no one did, unless it was very serious. The truth was, he frightened them, and they knew that his strength and power came from being apart from them. The tribe also knew that he did not live alone. He spoke to the fish, the animals, the birds, and the insects. Many said that he was able to communicate with the plants, the trees, the streams, and even the mist. He could tell the tribe when the snow or the lightning storms would come and, more important, where it was best to hunt the small animals and set the pitfalls for the larger ones. He was able to tell the tribe which roots, grains, berries, and nuts were good to eat and which plants could be used for medicine. The tribe believed their Shaman to be a powerful sorcerer.

Despite his heavy bearskin robe, the old man noiselessly entered the clearing downwind from the group gathered by the fire. As was his habit, when he got closer, he made enough noise to attract their attention without startling them. The members quickly turned and gave him a wide berth as he approached. They had urgently called him to cure a young man who had become very sick. The Shaman grimly approached the young man, who lay motionless on the soft bed of leaves and dried mulch. He knelt down and looked with regret upon the youthful face. He knew the boy well, because he was the one who the old man had chosen to be his replacement as the tribe's new

Shaman. His training had just begun, and the boy had proven to be a very intelligent and observant apprentice.

The frightened parents told the Shaman that the young man had returned from visiting the forest with his friends in the early afternoon. He had brought them back a fat marmot and was also carrying a sack full of acorns, berries, and mushrooms but had declined to eat with them because he and his friends had already done so. About an hour later, the boy began staggering around erratically, complaining of dizziness and terrible stomach pains. His parents tried feeding him, but he immediately vomited everything he ate. By the evening firelight, he started to get highly excited and frantically ran around the circle, from one member to the other, telling them of the grotesque monsters he had seen in the forest that day. His eyes opened wide, and his voice and motions hysterically portrayed the beasts that were coming to confront them. His agitation evolved into uncontrollable fits and convulsions before he finally collapsed, spots of white foam fringing the corners of his mouth. The tribe members became very frightened and immediately summoned the Shaman.

The old man placed his weathered hand upon the young man's cool, sweaty forehead and then bent over to smell the faint breath slowly issuing from his nostrils. He lifted the boy's hands and let them drop listlessly to the earth. After a few moments, the Shaman stood up and asked to see where the young man had vomited earlier. The boy's anxious mother picked a burning branch from the fire and led the old man to the spot. The Shaman slowly got down on all fours and asked the woman to hold the light close to the patch of damp earth so he could examine it more carefully. It didn't take long before he recognized what he was looking for. There, in the midst of the regurgitation, were small, grayish remnants of a warty mushroom cap, just as he had expected. Without giving any notice of his discovery, he quietly stood up and walked with the woman back to the others.

The Shaman adjusted his robe and took a pinch of dried herbs from one of the small leather pouches that hung from his waistband. He placed them in the palm of his hand and with the aid of some spit slowly rubbed them into a paste with his weathered index finger. Without any forewarning, he began to murmur a slow, rhythmical chant to the healing spirits of the forest. When the paste was the right consistency, he opened the boy's lips and smeared some of it onto his gums. The remaining material was rubbed onto the young man's forehead. The boy remained still. The Shaman stood up and continued to chant for a long time. Some of the tribe members, out of concern for the boy or simply overtaken by the sonorous rhythm of the chant, feebly joined in as best they could.

When he was through, the old man told the parents to cover the boy with a wolfskin robe and to continue their chanting throughout the night. If their worship was done with devotion, the boy would wake and return to normal by morning. The Shaman had done whatever magic was necessary to cure the boy—the rest was up to them. The young man's parents together with the remaining tribe members stooped respectfully and thanked the Shaman. As was their custom on his visits, they passed him a large sack of seeds, berries, and honeycombs that they had collected. The Shaman was a holy man—he never ate meat.

The Shaman took the sack and quickly faded into the forest. He again listened to all the familiar sounds as he walked in silence. He recalled the unending variety of shrubs and roots and flowers there were in the forest. He thought of all the food they provided his tribe and the animals. He also considered the plants that were used as powerful medicines and those that were dangerous to eat. A wise Shaman had to have such a vast store of knowledge to inform his people about the difference between plants that were good and those that were poisonous. The process of gaining this knowledge of good and evil was always demanding and occasionally dangerous.[1] There was so much to learn and so much to pass on to the next generations. He knew he had previously warned his protégé about that mushroom. He walked back to his lair with a troubled mind. There was a poisoner in the tribe!

NOTE

1. Muscimol is a potent neurotoxin produced by the Panthercap mushroom. This toxin has a rapid onset leading to tiredness, dizziness, and severe abdominal pain. Victims experience spells of excitability and hyperactivity, followed by delirium. Fatalities are not particularly common among adults, but it has been reported that young people may experience convulsions and comas for up to twelve hours.

INTRODUCTION

Looking after our health has always been a fundamental human preoccupation, which is understandable, since we are the only beings in the whole of the animal kingdom that are conscious of our own mortality.

From the methods and incantations of the shamans and witch doctors of our past to modern magnetic resonance imaging and emerging gene therapies, we've always tried to employ everything in our extensive arsenal of knowledge to forestall death and keep on living. While the recent advances in medical science have been truly amazing in extending the length of our lives, there is still much we do not know. In that sense, we are very much like our ancient forebears. They did not fully understand the basis of illness and usually attributed it to evil spirits of one form or another. They would kill and eat sick animals or scavenge carrion in complete ignorance of the disease-causing organisms they harbored. Even today, however, we have much to learn.

Traditionally, whenever issues of health or disease are discussed, we generally refer to the conditions that dominate the news, be it cancer, heart disease, or diabetes. In fact, this has been the case even when we talk about the effects of diet on health, as with cholesterol and cardiovascular disease, vegetable antioxidants and prostate cancer, or high-fiber diet and colon cancer. In the last few decades, however, another class of diseases directly related to the consumption of food has entered our common vocabulary—foodborne diseases. These are the diseases that are a direct result of eating accidentally— or deliberately—contaminated foods. More recently still, the specter of bioterrorism has raised its terrifying head, and the menace of a massive bio-based attack upon humankind through our food supplies is being considered very seriously—as it should be.

The recent spate of foodborne disease outbreaks has been a major concern to public health officials as well as consumers. Faced with the stress and uncertainty of this new challenge, it is not surprising that a great many people end up subscribing to the homespun theories of the back-to-earth or naturalist movement. But the medical and scientific communities both assure us that foodborne diseases are not new conditions. Foodborne diseases have been bedfellows of humankind from the dawn of creation.

Not unexpectedly, the assurances of the health professionals are based on the presumption that foodborne diseases are a phenomenon of nature—an integral part of the human condition. Many people, however, believe that these diseases are a unique result of modern, intensive agriculture and industrialized food processing. Scientists ask us to take a leap of faith and believe their theory, even though they have not provided to the general public any proof or evidence of these diseases in ancient times. This unsatisfying assertion spurs us to embark upon a voyage back in time to see what, if any, evidence exists to demonstrate that foodborne diseases have always been a challenge to us.

This trip back in time will not be a smooth journey through the continuum of human evolution but will be more like an exploration in a closed time capsule. We will be skipping back to distinct and separate periods, each one characterized by whatever evidence is available on foodborne disease. This is simply because foodborne diseases do not leave us with the same hard evidence, such as teeth and bones, which the evolutionary biologists rely on. As with any voyage of discovery, it would be best if we all understand what we are looking at. To make that task a little easier, let us put a few basics under our belts.

The term *disease* essentially defines itself—it literally means an absence of ease (dis-ease). When there is a clear means of identifying the manner in which a disease is transmitted to us, we categorize it. Thus, there are tick-borne diseases such as Lyme disease and Rocky Mountain spotted fever, as well as airborne diseases such as pneumonia, tuberculosis, and influenza. Of course, many other diseases result from metabolic imbalances or disturbances such as cardiovascular disease, or from pathogenic (disease-causing) biological agents. And, of course, there is cancer, which results from myriad causes, most of which remain to be elucidated.

The disease that is the subject of this book is "borne" to our bodies by the simple and routine act of consumption. Foodborne and waterborne diseases are those in which the pathogens are naturally present or have been intentionally placed in our food or beverages. Most often (but not always), foodborne and waterborne diseases result in some form of "gastroenteritis"—the irritation and inflammation of the gastrointestinal tract. The pathogenic agents causing the disease can be bacteria, toxins, molds, viruses, or parasites. In other cases, the agents can manifest themselves in more malignant forms of disease, such as severe neurological disorders and death.

The fact that the pathogenic agents enter our eating pathways and exert most of their effects on our soft tissues poses a real problem for the archaeologists and historians, not to mention the victims. Normally, the only things that can be dug up by archaeologists and paleontologists are objects that have survived the ages because they are hard and durable—rocks, shells, petrified wood, and, in the case of mammals, bones. Unfortunately, the symptoms of foodborne diseases are seldom displayed in skeletal remains. Foodborne and waterborne diseases exert their actions mainly upon soft tissues, so concrete evidence is extremely limited in prehistoric human remains.

All is not lost, however. Much may be learned through ancient paintings, hieroglyphics, or writings, which often depict life of prehistoric times in detailed ways. As time progressed and we developed writing as a means of expressing ourselves in a more exhaustive manner, improved historical records almost, in certain cases, obviated the need for physical evidence. For example, a careful examination of Socrates' skeletal remains would tell us very little about the manner of his death. But most researchers are fairly satisfied that the meticulous historical account of his suicide by drinking a cup of poison hemlock is valid. In addition to written records, both the intentional and the accidental means of preserving the bodies of the dead have provided a tremendous reserve of evidence of foodborne diseases. Mummification has resulted in bodies preserved so well that they are still useful for in-depth forensic examination. In these cases, we have the benefit of both written and some physical evidence.

So, despite the limited amount of what many might consider hard data, a great deal of evidence of credible quality can be used to get a reasonable perspective on the role of foodborne and waterborne diseases in history.

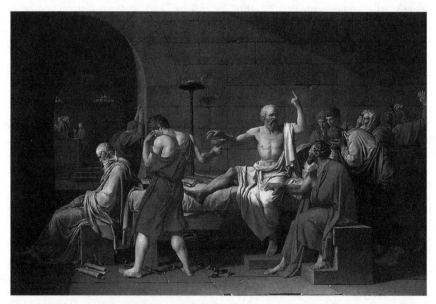

The Death of Socrates, oil on canvas by Jacques-Louis David, 1787, in the Metropolitan Museum of Art, New York City. B/W photo by M. Satin.

WHAT EVIDENCE IS THERE OF FOODBORNE DISEASES IN ANTIQUITY?

Most of us are familiar with the term *pathology*, the study of diseases. Paleopathology is simply the study of diseases in ancient times. From a practical point of view, it is the science of studying the evidence of disease on ancient remains. The term *ancient* is somewhat subjective and extends over a rather long period of time, from prehistoric to near contemporary times (frequently considered to be the fall of the Western Roman Empire, 476 CE), and thus covers such evidence as skeletal remains, mummies, and bog bodies.

Although there are many modern methods used in the field of pale-opathology, the most important is the traditional one—close visual observation. The changes that can be seen in bones usually indicate how an individual reacted to a physical challenge, predicament, or disease over a long period of time. Even the way that new bone tissue was formed can provide the paleopathologist with evidence of certain disease conditions. On the other hand, the absence of abnormalities on the skeletal remains does not mean that the individual was free of disease. It only means that if there was disease, it did not affect the bones.

Equally important to the paleopathologist is an understanding of the population dynamics that took place during the period under study. This, together with the physical evidence—and, wherever possible, historical accounts—provides an idea of the relative importance of diseases and their impact on the society. During the general course of history, population growth has been fairly steady. The only periods of exceptional growth were those that followed major technological innovations, such as the agricultural and industrial revolutions.

BONES AND BONES

Obviously, skeletons and skulls can only show evidence of diseases that leave their marks upon bone. Thus, a great number of diseases that exclusively affect the soft tissues are not accounted for. In some cases, however, soft tissue diseases are of a long-term chronic nature with secondary effects that can eventually appear on the skeleton. Thus, crippling nervous disorders start out as soft tissue diseases (brain and nervous system) but in time show their effects upon the bones, because the musculoskeletal system can no longer function as originally intended and the bones become marked or deformed.

Nevertheless, most soft tissue diseases do not show symptoms upon the skull or skeleton. In the case of foodborne or waterborne diseases, the symptoms are usually acute (intense and short term) rather then chronic (long term), which doesn't leave enough time to exert an obvious impact upon the bones. One exception is the recently discovered evidence that certain foodborne disease organisms can have long-term aftereffects, or sequelae. Specifically, it has been found that foodborne infections of the bacteria *Campylobacter*, the most common foodborne disease organism, can result in reactive arthritis long after the gastroenteritis symptoms are gone. The bacteria exert their acute effects in the intestine, exacting on their victims a short-term incidence of diarrhea, headache, and fever, which is gone in a few days. However, the same bacteria can also invade the largest joints and exert long-term chronic effects eventually leading to crippling arthritis, long after any memories of the original gastrointestinal incident have disappeared.

Although the evidence of disease that exists on skeletal remains is fairly limited, modern chemical and physical analysis can provide some idea of the disease conditions and challenges faced by the various societies in the past. Bones derived from skeletons excavated in archaeological studies show a great range of pathological conditions. These can include abnormal bone growth owing to arthritis or worn-away lesions, reflecting bacterial infections or other stressful conditions. These skeletal remains can provide significant information, suggesting the diseases that ancient people suffered. Some chronic disorders such as stunted growth from starvation or rickets from malnutrition are also ascertainable from evidence on long leg bones.

The most obvious evidence exhibited by bones results from trauma such as breaks, fractures, dislocation complications, and deformities. In other instances, gaping holes can be found in skulls, the result of fighting or acts of war. In still other cases, skulls show clear evidence of scalping —an old practice for collecting trophies from a vanquished enemy.

One of the oddities found in skulls are "trepanation" holes. Trepanation is an ancient practice and is still carried out today in isolated primitive societies. It is the forerunner of neurosurgery and involves making an incision in the scalp followed by the removal of a piece of skull. The idea is to expose the brain membranes to the open air for a period of time. It is a wonder that anyone was able to survive this horrendous procedure— but survive they did, since there is evidence of healing in a large percentage of ancient skulls found with trepanation holes.

It is likely that the major reason for trepanation was to allow the evil spirits—which were thought to be responsible for migraine headaches or other severe head pains—to escape. Needless to say, we all owe a great debt of gratitude to Dr. Bayer for his discovery of the means of commercially producing aspirin.

Evidence of joint disorders is fairly common in ancient skeletons, including various forms of arthritis, particularly osteoarthritis owing to age, physical stress, and genetic disposition—much the same as today. Often osteoarthritis evidence can provide clues to the occupation of the individual and the type of society that he or she lived in. It is possible, for instance, to tell the difference between a hunter-gatherer and a farmer through the manner in which each occupation exerted physical stress on the various bones of the individual.

EVIDENCE IN TEETH

Surprisingly, although dental cavities were common in prehistoric animals such as fish, reptiles, and mammals, most early humans have shown limited evidence of this problem. In fact, cavities began to be manifest in humans only after fermentable sugars became a regular part of the diet.

Although there is limited evidence of dental cavities in our ancestors, there is significant evidence of wear on tooth surfaces because of the abrasive nature of the foods consumed, particularly after agriculture became a mainstay of our diet. All the grain that was ground in stone mills contained small fragments of stone and sand, which wore away the teeth. The same can be said for the consumption of other products taken from the soil, such as roots and tubers. Soil and sand particles adhere to foods, and since our forebears were not too fastidious about washing them off, the inevitable result was abnormally high tooth wear. In fact, you can still find this phenomenon today in communities where small seeds such as millet and sorghum are staples in the daily diet. The dirt and grit are just too laborious to remove completely, so it is consumed with the grain. Some other habits, such as chewing betel nuts, also led to abnormally high tooth wear—a characteristic that continues to be seen in many developing countries today.

COPROLITES

Desiccated feces or intestinal contents are formally known as coprolites (aka paleopoop) and can be one of the archaeologist's most valuable artifacts, particularly if foodborne diseases are the object of study. Almost no foods are digested completely, and coprolites contain the remnants of the diet as well as the remains of pathogenic organisms. Whereas soft tissue cannot generally survive through the ages, coprolites can, and the microorganisms they contain are often robust enough to remain intact throughout the centuries. Fortunately for the archaeologist, many societies had common areas (latrines) for holding feces, so the samples found there often represent the general spectrum of society at large. The resulting coprolite material has been invaluable in demonstrating the type of diets people enjoyed as well as the foodborne parasites that ancient societies, both the rich and the poor, endured. (These parasites will be referred to later in this book.)

MUMMIES

Among the most valuable remains available to those who study diseases in antiquity are mummies. Although mummies are usually identified with the ancient Egyptians—those that were embalmed and wrapped in swaddling strips of cloth—the term *mummy* is more broadly defined to cover all well-preserved ancient bodies. Such bodies are often found in dry places such as deserts or dry caves, or in high mountainous altitudes, such as the Andes, which are also very dry. The dry, cold low-pressure atmospheres typical of these altitudes act very much like an efficient freeze-dryer to desiccate and preserve bodies perfectly.

The ancient process of preservation of Egyptian mummies is no longer a secret. In the same way that many foods are preserved, salt was used as the drying agent in the Egyptians' standard mummification process, prior to the complex wrapping of the bodies. The salting process was supplemented with tar or pitch, as well as oils and resins to prevent the rehydration of the tissues. In fact, the term *mummy* comes from the Persian word *mumeia*, which literally means "pitch."

There are also mummies from China that have been preserved in excellent condition because the mercury-based embalming solutions prevented natural decomposition and also destroyed any contaminating microorganisms. To further ensure protection of the bodies, the coffins were hermetically sealed to completely exclude oxygen.

Perfectly preserved bodies are also found in the permafrost. As a result of the low ambient temperatures, these bodies simply froze and remained that way until uncovered.

BOG BODIES

Among the most interesting preserved bodies that are of historical interest are bog bodies. In the past, almost all bog bodies were recovered from northwest Europe, but more recently, they have been found in the bogs of central Europe as well as in the British Isles. These bodies were preserved as a result of natural phenomena rather than a purposeful attempt at preservation, as was the case with the Egyptian mummies. A typical bog is a standing body of water with a great deal of organic matter from trees and plants and no underground spring of fresh water to feed and replenish it. The water is generally cold, extremely acidic (because of the broken-down inorganic material), low in oxygen, and loaded with tannic substances—all told, an ideal environment for embalming bodies. As a result, these bodies are very well preserved and are able to provide substantial information on food habits, lifestyles, diseases, and chronic toxins.

With all well-preserved bodies, forensic examinations can be made of the tissues in order to understand the body's pathology. In addition to the soft tissues such as muscles, other tissues such as hair and nails can be very useful. Nails and hair can absorb toxic substances such as arsenic and bind it tightly. Since these tissues grow slowly, they accumulate and hold onto these toxins with the result that evidence of poisoning can remain for eons.

THE ANALYSIS OF EVIDENCE

Finding evidence of ancient people is just the beginning. Once the evidence is discovered, various analyses have to be carried out, such as ascertaining who the individual might have been, what society he or she belonged to, how he and his family lived, and finally, how he died. People very often die of causes not necessarily connected to the chronic diseases or conditions that they suffered from on a day-to-day basis.

As mentioned earlier, simple skeletal evidence is of very limited value in the study of foodborne diseases. However, mummies offer an extended scope of evidence related to diseases that are soft tissue–based. Aside from visual examination, tissues can be chemically analyzed to determine their mineral components, and even the DNA can be examined to look at genetic origins. In scientists' search of historical evidence, mummies have gone through the entire repertoire of modern medical tests and analyses that any person would have if being examined by a doctor for any variety of diseases.

Ancient food and water sources can be estimated through the analysis and microscopic examination of stomach and intestinal contents as well as the mineral contents of the soft tissues. Careful microscopic analysis can also reveal evidence of pathogenic organisms such as molds and parasites.

More recently, the modern techniques of molecular biology have been put to work in analyzing ancient remains. The new discipline of paleogenetics seeks to characterize the DNA of ancient remains in order to determine their genetic origins. Very small amounts of genetic material can be used to identify both natural and foreign or infectious DNA. This can provide clear evidence of certain diseases. As an example, the DNA from the bacteria responsible for tuberculosis was recently extracted from a thousand-year-old Peruvian mummy.[1]

Perhaps the most productive area of study for evidence of food-borne diseases in ancient remains is the study of diet and the investigation of intestinal and fecal materials, whenever they are available. Over the years, sophisticated forensic techniques have been developed to precisely identify a wide range of materials found in diets such as fruit seeds, marine shells, pollen, grains, and bone fragments.

In addition to the actual body remains, it is also possible to get evidence of diets from the area surrounding the burial site itself, since foods were often interred along with the corpses. Some of the best examples of this are the tombs of the ancient Egyptian mummies, which usually contained copious amounts of foods well preserved in sealed vessels. It was believed that food should accompany the body to nourish it in its long journey through the afterlife.

The analysis of intestinal contents is particularly valuable, since they reflect the residues of the individual's last meals. These materials along with coprolites can be gently broken down to reveal all the components of the individual's diet. In fact, specific food plants can be determined from leaf fragments or even the size and shape of single-starch granules.

Fish scales or mollusk shells can indicate the kind of marine diet that was consumed and whether the individuals went out to sea or collected their food from the shoreline. Small bones can be associated with the types of birds or small mammals that were part of their everyday diet and could be found in the surrounding area.

Initially, coprolite analysis was limited to the study of mummified remains, but more recently, large communal waste pits and latrines have been found and analyzed to provide evidence of diet and disease in large communities. In one of the more interesting instances, such analyses were recently carried out on the palatial remains of one of history's most glittering monarchs (to be discussed later).

As coprolite analysis became increasingly more sophisticated, it was possible to accurately determine some of the pathogenic organisms that infected ancient people. All stages of parasite infection from eggs to larvae to adults have been found, often in very large quantities. Being able to analyze down to the species level can also provide evidence of migration of diseases, for if a parasite is not native or endemic to a particular region, it is likely to have been brought there through visitation or migration from other regions.

Ancient societies suffered terribly from a great many parasites. Egyptian mummies were found with beef and pork tapeworms, liver flukes, whipworms, guinea worms, huge intestinal roundworms, *Trichinella*, *Ascaris*, and many other foodborne and waterborne parasites. Even though the Egypt of the pharaohs was considered to be a grand and highly sophisticated nation, the hygienic and sanitation practices were very poor. Consequently, parasite eggs shed in the feces reentered the infection cycle through the food and water and continually plagued all classes of the population.

Despite the large amount of evidence that is available through paleopathology, enormous gaps in our knowledge continue to frustrate us. In many cases, there is almost no physical evidence at all of certain societies, yet we are certain of their existence through historical writings. Without direct physical evidence, the most productive way to gain a perspective on the lives of ancient people is to reread the historical accounts and interpret them in light of the knowledge that we have accumulated since they were originally written.

THE MASS OF EVIDENCE
FROM HISTORICAL ACCOUNTS

Because the physical evidence of disease throughout history is so limited, we must rely heavily on other evidence to supplement our knowledge. From the earliest time, humans have kept records of their lives and their interactions with others and the environment. Thus, we have many primitive pictorial works, highly artistic representations, petroglyphs, complex hieroglyphics, and written-language records that can provide information on ancient people, how they lived, and what they ate.

The list of such materials available to us is impressive. Rock paintings and rock carvings made by primitive ancestors can be found on every continent as well as from the Arctic to the South Pacific. The images, painted or etched on rocks, in caves or under overhanging cliffs, describe the artist's environment, including pictures of the local plants and animals as well as the people. Some of the images created are almost fifteen thousand years old, yet they retain a magical and fluid beauty. From these paintings we can learn not only what people ate but also about their experiences in obtaining food. More recent findings have revealed cave paintings in Italy that are reported to be thirty-five thousand years old![2]

It is not known exactly who invented writing, but it probably originated around 6000 BCE. The art of writing developed independently in Egypt, Mesopotamia, China, and Central America. Most people are familiar with hieroglyphics, the pictorial form of writing used in ancient Egypt. Similar forms of writing are found in Crete, Central America, and Mexico. Hieroglyphics were used to represent words and concepts. They were pieced together to relate stories and to form a historical record of the times. Such records often describe the diet, the way foods were prepared, and the diseases that affected the people of the time.

Cuneiform writing was developed by the Sumerians around the same time that hieroglyphics were invented (4000 BCE). This writing is made up of thin, wedge-shaped strokes impressed upon clay tablets, then baked for permanency. Alphabetic systems date from about 1500 BCE; around 800 BCE, the Greeks took the final step by separating the vowels and consonants to arrive at full alphabetic writing.

The most celebrated work in writing in the Western world is the Bible. Genesis was first written in the tenth century BCE, with the remaining books of the Old Testament completed within the suc-ceeding millennium. The Old Testament has several references to foods, their consumption, prohibitions, and the pathological condi-tions that could result from improper consumption. Indeed, the very first law stated in the Bible is a food law. In Genesis, chapter 2, verses 16 and 17, it is stated: "And the Lord God commanded the man, saying, of every tree of the garden thou mayest freely eat; but of the tree of the knowledge of good and evil, thou shalt not eat of it: for in the day that thou eateth thereof thou shalt surely die."

In Leviticus, chapter 12, God clearly describes in great detail the animals that were permitted to be consumed. A cursory review of the list is interesting because it describes both the physical and sacro-social reasons for prohibition. The list describes several personal sanitation and hygiene practices to follow in order to remain pure and clean. It is really quite amazing how close these practices come to those that are used today. From the time such rules were first written until the basic concepts of hygiene were scientifically verified, most societies were totally ignorant of these practices and did not follow them. Primitive societies today still do not follow these practices, yet there they were, clearly prescribed more than three thousand years ago.

Chapter 15 of Leviticus describes illnesses in people and how such illnesses are to be considered elements of uncleanliness. It illustrates the phenomenon of contamination and goes on to describe the neces-sity to clean and wash those who are ill. With very little rewriting, Leviticus's words can be used as a guideline for hygiene practices today.

Egyptian hieroglyphics described many of the foods consumed in the country during the days of the pharaohs. Even though there were prohibitions against certain foods, such as pork, it appears elsewhere that those foods were consumed. In fact, some hieroglyphics describe regulations that were enforced to control the consumption of prohibited foods.

By the time we arrive at the glory of ancient Greece, the writings have evolved to a highly detailed record not unlike modern chronicles. The ancient Greeks and Romans also spent a considerable amount of time describing food consumption habits and, in some cases, food poisoning in their writings. Hippocrates, Horace, and Ovid all wrote about the poisonous effects of mushrooms and other plants. As an example, history records that poisonous mushrooms tragically destroyed the entire family of the Greek poet Euripides.

The Greek philosopher Theophrastus made many references to poisons in his book on plants, including those used to intentionally poison people. Xenophon states that intentional poisoning was so common that tasters were employed to check foods before they were presented to royalty—a practice that continued for two thousand years! The Greek and Roman writers also went to lengths to describe the practice of food adulteration—a trend first started from the time that foods and food ingredients became items of trade.

During the medieval period, records show that accidental and intentional food poisonings along with food adulterations were commonplace. Diseased animals were slaughtered and, together with animals that had previously succumbed to disease, were treated with adulterants to hide any evidence of their poor quality—a practice that is still carried out by unscrupulous operators today. One of the most popular uses of the newly discovered spice nutmeg was to hide the smell and taste of spoiled meat. The taste of nutmeg became so common and so closely associated with meat that even today it is the main spice used in hot dogs and sausages.

Despite the overriding influence of religion upon medieval life, it is clear that the precepts of hygiene, so beautifully detailed in

Leviticus, were never spoken of by the clergy. Regardless of the common expression that "cleanliness is next to Godliness," cleanliness had no apparent place or priority in medieval religion.[3] The hygienic conditions of slaughterhouses and other food preparation premises as well as those of the home and castle were abhorrent by today's standards and remained that way until the dawn of the twentieth century.

From the sixteenth century onward, a scientific understanding of the origin and basis of diseases slowly began to be established. This resulted in a growing number of publications in the scientific and technical literature specifically focused on the subject of disease. These documents are interesting because they displaced the variety of interpretations made of evidence until a definitive and undisputed answer was eventually found. The annals of science are littered with the remains of quack theories and equally useless treatments that were proffered up until something that passed objective scientific scrutiny was eventually discovered.

How fortunate we are that so many accounts describing everyday existence became part of the historical record. Scientific reports, city records, ships' logs, legal transcripts, and even novels and theatrical performances all contained descriptions of everyday life and serve as excellent sources of information regarding the diseases or conditions that afflicted our forebears.

Despite the fact that the individuals writing the historical record were unaware of the actual disease that the symptoms they recorded reflected, their historical accounts were often so detailed that, in light of our present knowledge, it is possible to say with near certainty what the diseases they described actually were.

At other times, we can only speculate on the real nature of the evidence presented, as, for example, with the Salem witch trials. The witch theory prevalent at the time was based on a dogmatic fundamentalist belief. There was neither the knowledge nor the will to seek explanations for the witches' behavior elsewhere. (In case we feel so much more sophisticated and progressive than our Puritan ancestors, we should not forget that the initial discovery of the HIV virus and

AIDS was greeted by some fundamentalist church folk with the theory that it was not a biological problem but rather a punishment by God for immoral behavior.)

Taken together, the physical and historical evidence tells us that foodborne disease has been a constant companion of humankind throughout history. As we shall see, diseases have been associated with some of the most dramatic episodes of history, even though the victims were totally unaware of their presence. Lacking the wisdom and discipline to forsake all forms of edible temptation, our first ancestors foolishly tasted of the tree of knowledge of good and evil. They were unceremoniously banished from the Garden of Eden and commenced their long journey down through the ages. Let's follow along and discover some of the other edible temptations that proved impossible to resist.

NOTES

1. S. Pääbo et al., "Genetic Analyses from Ancient DNA," *Annual Review of Genetics* 38 (2004): 645–79.

2. Anonymous, "Oldest Cave Paintings Ever Found Light Up Human History," *Guardian Unlimited*, October 19, 2000, http://www.asa3.org/archive/ASA/200010/0300.html (accessed October 4, 2005).

3. In his book *Advancement of Learning*, published in 1605, Francis Bacon wrote: "Cleanness of body was ever deemed to proceed from a due reverence to God."

PART I
THE ANCIENT WORLD

CHAPTER 1
THE HEBREWS AND EGYPTIANS
(4000 BCE–100 CE)

PREHISTORY

T he period of history before the appearance of written records is generally referred to as prehistory. This includes the Stone Age, the Bronze Age, and the Iron Age—times when many societies did manage to preserve their histories but through an oral tradition of folktales and stories passed on from generation to generation. If, for some reason, the society vanished, so did all remnants of its history unless enough archaeological evidence was left behind for a cohesive record to be pieced together.

The Stone Age was that period of time before the use of basic metals, when all hard tools, implements, and weapons were fashioned from stone. The dates of the Stone Age vary from one part of the world to another, but it is generally agreed that it began about two million years ago in Asia, Africa, and Europe and ended in Southeast Asia and the Middle East about eight thousand years ago. However, remnants of it lingered on for another two thousand years in Europe, Africa, and the rest of Asia. In the New World of the Americas, the Stone Age began about thirty thousand years ago, when humans first arrived there, and ended about four thousand years ago.

Throughout the Stone Age, immense changes took place in the environment, which significantly affected the evolution and development of human culture. Because of the fundamental transformations that took place, the Stone Age is divided into three distinct stages of development, namely, the Paleolithic, Mesolithic, and Neolithic periods.

The Paleolithic period, which initiated the Stone Age, began when the first humanoids started using stone tools and ended at the closing stages of the last ice age, about fifteen thousand years ago. Life was sustained through hunting and gathering, and evidence of these humanoids' culture survives chiefly through the remains of very basic stone tools, which along with carbon dating can be used to determine the chronology of their existence. Handheld scalloped stone tools were used for digging up roots in hard soils, for killing small animals, and for crudely skinning and cutting up carcasses. Over an extended period of time, the variety of tools improved, as did their degree of sophistication needed to cope with the changing demands of life. Other materials such as bone were used to fashion the sewing needles required for making the clothes needed to survive the colder weather or for fishing hooks to help expand the sources of food available.

About five hundred thousand years ago, a new immigrant population, *Homo heidelbergensis*, with excellent hunting skills, as evidenced by its advanced weapons such as spears, firmly established itself in Europe. This group eventually gave rise to the Neanderthals— burly, big-brained humans with short arms and a broad trunk, who appeared in Europe about two hundred and fifty thousand years ago.

The Neanderthal people of the period roamed over parts of Europe and the Middle East. Their time was one of great hardship, with less than half the population surviving to the age of twenty, and virtually no one living beyond forty years. It was a time when the continual shortages of food led to widespread malnutrition and routine seasonal starvation. A desperate attempt to seek out anything that looked the least bit edible and a very limited understanding of plant toxicity resulted in many debilitating illnesses or deaths. The same result occurred after the consumption of toxic or contaminated fish or meat.

Around the same time that the Neanderthals developed, a new African group, *Homo sapiens*, spread to Asia, continued to evolve, and eventually trekked north to Europe as Cro-Magnons. This group had a larger cranial capacity than modern humans and were quite capable of intuitive thinking. Neanderthals and Cro-Magnons came in contact with each other around two hundred thousand years ago and probably coexisted for several thousand years. However, this encounter with *H. sapiens*, our direct forebears, was of no benefit to the Neanderthals, who ultimately disappeared about twenty-five thousand to thirty thousand years ago.

The Mesolithic period, or Middle Stone Age, started about ten thousand to fifteen thousand years ago with the end of the glacial period. The milder weather had the positive effect of making a greater and more varied food supply available. The retreat of glaciers and the consequent growth of forests in Europe allowed Mesolithic cultures to enjoy a much wider variety of food from hunting, fishing, and gathering activities. Fishing settlements appeared along lake and river shores where fish and shellfish were readily available. Archaeological studies have unearthed large deposits of mollusk shells around these settlements. This period was characterized by an abundance of newly available plant species that were gradually domesticated along with the animals that lived in proximity to settlements. By "domesticated," I mean acclimatized to deliberate cultivation.

Mesolithic tools, still fairly primitive, were adapted to the new environmental conditions and became smaller and more refined. It was during this period that hafted axes (where the axe blade is bound tightly to the wood shaft) were developed—a great improvement over the handheld stone axe of the Paleolithic period. The bow and arrow was also developed, which greatly increased the efficiency of hunting and gave access to a much wider variety of animal foods. The Mesolithic period was one of significant technical and social evolution, and the continual quest for an easier and more secure existence evolved into the Neolithic period, the final phase of the Stone Age.

The most important change to characterize the Neolithic period was the much greater role that agriculture assumed in providing a stable supply of food. The earliest evidence of the shift from a Mesolithic to a Neolithic way of life occurred in the Middle East, where agricultural villages began to develop about ten thousand years ago. These generally began as settlements located near fields offering abundant supplies of wild grains. Eventually, it was discovered that grain that accidentally spilled onto the ground grew into mature plants that provided grain the following year. The rudimentary seeds of modern agriculture were sown—perhaps the greatest evolutionary episode in the history of human civilization.

A stable and reliable supply of food meant that humans were able to spend more time doing things other than hunting and gathering. Pottery soon appeared, and not long after, copper began to be used in jewelry making and toolmaking in some regions. The Bronze and Iron Ages followed in fairly quick succession.

It is difficult to say precisely which foodborne diseases our Stone Age ancestors suffered from, because there is no direct evidence or records available. However, we can assume with some confidence that they regularly ate contaminated meat and fish, poisonous mushrooms, toxic plants, and raw, indigestible grains. Notwithstanding their hardy constitutions and continual exposure to a variety of contaminating organisms, it is likely that they routinely suffered, and often died from, gastrointestinal-related diseases.

Unfortunately, there is a limit to the hard evidence available regarding the foods our forebears ate. If a roasted leg of mastodon happened to be on the menu, the chances of finding prehistoric evidence of that particular meal would be much better than if the meal was a few baby quails. Small animals, the ones most likely to be consumed, leave virtually no archaeological evidence. The same can be said for most plant materials. Whatever was not digested was eventually ground together with all other organic and inorganic materials into dust. The fact that our ancient ancestors were nomadic presumes that they were hunters and scroungers and consumed whatever they could in one area. And when that was exhausted, they simply moved on.

Until the advent of fire, there was no means of limiting the bacterial contamination of foods. The first strong evidence that fire was used to heat or cook foods comes from the Zhoukoudian caves in China. Here, four hundred thousand years ago, *Homo erectus* was able to use fire to roast meat on the bone to make it softer or tastier. By the time of Neanderthal man, cooking to improve palatability was carried out by boiling food in water held in leather vessels into which heated stones had been placed. It was a primitive and not overly effective way of reducing contamination, but it was a beginning.

The variety of foods consumed by primitive humans was highly varied and dependent upon their geographic location, the time of year, and the degree of organization of their societies. Well-organized groups could have hunted and eaten buffalo, bear, moose, or other large animals in North America. In the Asia-Pacific region, the same sorts of groups could have taken down bears, wild pigs, water buffaloes, monkeys, and even elephants. In the wilds of Russia, mountain goats, horses, bears, and leopards could have been on the menu, while in Africa, elephant, rhinoceros, zebra, kudu, lion, leopard, hyena, and porcupine were consumed.

Less-organized groups or individuals could not be quite so ambitious and had to settle for smaller beasts, including rats, hares, mice, squirrels, lemurs, beavers, and raccoons. Of course, insects, snails, shellfish, and a great variety of plants, tree nuts, mushrooms, fruits, and roots were eaten whenever and wherever they could be found.

It would be logical to assume that these people suffered regularly from the widest possible range of foodborne illnesses. Like all other predators, they consumed the sickest or weakest animals because they were the easiest to kill. They also ate putrid meat that had been hidden away for long periods as well as noxious plants or mushrooms. While some societies may have grown more tolerant to certain toxic or other pathogenic challenges, most of our prehistoric ancestors generally died in poor health at an age of twenty to thirty years. The good old days were not very good, and people rarely grew old.

REVOLUTION THROUGH EVOLUTION

Looking back through history, we have a tendency to consider major changes in our lifestyles and social habits as revolutionary. In truth, these changes occurred very slowly. The development of farming did not take place in one generation or over one century, it took place gradually over *millennia*. The individuals who spilled the grain one year were not the ones who found the seedlings growing the following year and concluded that there might be good business prospects in this development. Settlements occurred around seedlings long before anyone made a connection between them and previously spilled grain. But growing settlements did mean more spilled grains and the seedlings that resulted from them, so agriculture was eventually learned and adopted almost by accident.

The development of agriculture occurred repeatedly and independently in various parts of the world, after the retreat of the glaciers around twelve thousand years ago. The warming trend affected China, the Middle East, and Central America, where agriculture began in earnest. The availability of a consistent supply of foods such as grains reduced the need of going farther and farther afield to find food, and nomadic wandering was gradually reduced. Decreasing the pressure on the local wildlife resulted in the wildlife multiplying and being attracted to the settlements where any excess food became an easy meal.

With time, animals became familiar enough with people to enter into a form of domestication for the mutual benefit of both. Beginning with dogs, followed by sheep, goats, pigs, and finally cattle, a whole range of animals eventually became part of a settlement's entourage. This relationship often started with feeding and petting and ended with a whack on the head and a quick toss onto the communal cooking pit. Dogs eventually were spared this fate because they were more valuable as camp guardians, they were unusually loyal to their masters, and, most important, they were quick and had very sharp teeth. Sheep, on the other hand, presented no such dilemma. (Many societies continue to enjoy "man's best friend," at least the more manageable varieties, up to the present time.)

The Neolithic period (seven thousand to ten thousand years ago) is characterized by the use of advanced stone tools, permanent villages, advances in pottery making and weaving, and increased domestication of animals and plants. Thus, the domestication of food animals developed in parallel with the beginnings of organized agriculture. This was not so much a revolution as an evolution of customs with people using their growing intellectual capacity to slowly develop the means of achieving a sustainable livelihood while remaining in one location. It matters not whether agriculture as we know it first developed along the Indus River or the Fertile Crescent running from the Nile Valley to the Tigris and Euphrates rivers, what is important is that the entire lifestyle of people changed as a result of the adoption of agriculture.

ANCIENT EGYPT

Egyptian history can be traced back through an uninterrupted six-thousand-year-old record depicted in the paintings of tombs and burial chambers. This evidence, which we're fortunate to have, demonstrates that ancient Egypt was the source of a significant part of the agricultural technology that developed in the Western world.

The types of crops the ancient Egyptians cultivated can be seen in their artistic renditions as well as the organic remains of plants retrieved from tombs. The major staples were ancient grain crops, roots, various legumes, cucumbers, melons, and salads. Garlic and onions were also very popular. Among the favorite fruits were dates, figs, grapes, pomegranates, apples, and olives.

The ancient Egyptians distinguished between two different categories of domesticated animals, large and small. Large cattle consisted essentially of cows and bulls, while pigs, goats, and sheep fell into the small category. Cows were also used for the production of milk. Based on the archaeological evidence available, it is clear that both wild and

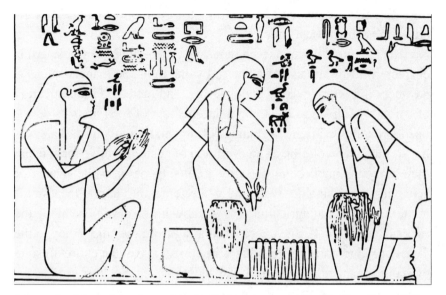

Hieroglyphic taken from N. de G. Davies and A. H. Gardiner, "The Tomb of Antifoker," Egypt Exploration Society (London: George Allen and Unwin, 1920).

domesticated pigs were consumed in great numbers. In addition, the bones of various antelopes, gazelles, horses, and donkeys have been found in burial sites throughout Egypt, indicating that these animals were consumed whenever available.

Fermentation was discovered and used in the production of bread and wine. Grain was ground in a small stone hand mill, made into dough, and allowed to ferment naturally. The natural yeast leaven was saved from batch to batch to improve and speed up subsequent bread-making efforts. The hieroglyph above depicts the production of bread in shaped molds.[1]

Liquid fermentation was carried out in clay vessels using the same yeast source as bread. The result was beer if the liquid mash was based on grain, and wine if the original liquid came from fruit juice. Grapes made a particularly good wine and came with their own supply of fermentation yeast on their skins.

Although the ancient Egyptians enjoyed a highly varied diet, which was well described through their record of hieroglyphics, there are not many descriptions related to foodborne or waterborne diseases. The few that are available appear to be more broadly described in the biblical record.

THE BIBLICAL RECORD

The first instance of God's word being written down, according to the Bible, was the Ten Commandments delivered to Moses in the form of stone tablets on Mount Sinai about thirty-five hundred years ago. The original scriptures are generally considered to be the first five books of the Bible—Genesis, Exodus, Leviticus, Numbers, and Deuteronomy —collectively called the Pentateuch. Written in an ancient form of Hebrew on sheepskin scrolls, the full Pentateuch is called a Torah and was passed down from generation to generation.

By approximately 500 BCE, the thirty-nine books that make up the Old Testament were completed and continued to be preserved in Hebrew on scrolls. In the last few centuries before Christ, the Jewish historical books known as the Apocrypha were completed; however, they were recorded in Greek rather than Hebrew. By the end of the first century CE, the New Testament had been completed. It was preserved in Greek on papyrus, a thin paperlike material made from crushed and flattened stalks of a reedlike plant. The word *Bible* comes from the same Greek root word as *papyrus*. The papyrus sheets were bound or tied together in a configuration much more similar to modern books than to an extended scroll.

Based upon descriptions in the Bible, the foods available to the ancient Hebrews were generally similar to those of the ancient Egyptians. The main differences in consumption patterns between the two peoples resulted from the strict prohibitions enshrined in the Jewish dietary laws.

As previously mentioned, it is interesting that the very first law quoted in the Bible is a dietary law. From Genesis:

2:16. God gave the man a commandment, saying, "You may definitely eat from every tree of the garden."

2:17. But from the Tree of Knowledge of good and evil, do not eat, for on the day you eat from it, you will definitely die.[2]

The reference to "every tree of the garden" makes it clear that God intended us to be vegetarians. This is further confirmed by a previous passage:

1:29. God said, "Behold, I have given you every seedbearing plant on the face of the earth, and every tree that has seedbearing fruit. It shall be to you for food."

1:30. For every beast of the field, every bird of the sky, and everything that walks the land, that has in it a living soul, all plant vegetation shall be food. It remained that way.[3]

To refrain from killing and consuming animals was an ethical decision. However, it was not long before the foibles and malice of human character became apparent, giving God cause to regret his greatest creation. From Genesis:

6:5. God saw that man's wickedness on earth was increasing. Every impulse of his innermost thought was only for evil, all day long.

6:6. God regretted that He had made man on earth, and He was pained to His very core.

6:7. God said, "I will obliterate humanity that I have created from the face of the earth—man, livestock, land animals, and birds of the sky. I regret that I created them."

6:8. But Noah found favor in God's eyes.[4]

With the exception of Noah, his family, and the animals on board the ark, all life was destroyed by the Great Flood. It was the beginning of a new civilization, and it was only then that God relented and permitted Noah and all his dependents to eat the meat of animals.

9:3. Every moving thing that lives shall be to you as food. Like plant vegetation, I have now given you everything.[5]

The permission to eat meat appeared to be the result of God's diminished expectations of mankind, a concession to man's animal nature. But this was not given without conditions, for the verse immediately following sets out the first stricture on blood consumption that served as the basis of the Jewish dietary laws.

9:4. But nevertheless, you may not eat flesh of a creature that is still alive.

Contrary to popular belief, the Jewish dietary laws were not based on any known relationship between diet and disease. The only purpose for the kosher laws was to aspire to holiness and perfection by emphasizing certain moral and ethical obligations. The permitted animals were slaughtered quickly and with the least amount of pain inflicted. Only clean and healthy animals were consumed, because anything else was considered unfit if one was to maintain a sense of spiritual purity. Once an animal was slaughtered, it was forbidden to consume its blood, because that was where the soul of the animal was considered to reside. An uppermost objective of these practices was the differentiation of humans from all other animals. Pigs were not consumed simply because they were considered dirty and represented some of the basest habits in the animal kingdom, not because it was known that they harbored diseases such as trichinosis.

Despite the moral and ethical basis for their promulgation, the Jewish dietary laws also happened to make good hygienic sense, and the ancient Hebrews who strictly followed them generally suffered from fewer gastrointestinal diseases than their neighbors.

Within the Pentateuch, however, a number of foodborne and waterborne poisoning incidents are depicted. Even though much of the text is allegorical in nature, both the circumstances and the symptoms are described in sufficient detail to allow a credible disease diagnosis to be made. Even more important is the fact that identical poisonings have occurred in the same geographical region for millennia and still occur today.

EVENT 1. A TALE OF QUAIL

One of the greatest epics narrated in the Bible is the book of Exodus, which describes the flight of the Hebrews from Egypt and their wanderings through the desert to Mount Sinai in the "Promised Land." Exodus describes the oppression of the Hebrews by the Egyptians, the birth of Moses, his selection by God to lead the Hebrews out of Egypt, the ten plagues brought upon the Egyptians, the narrow escape from Egypt, and the forty years of wandering through the desert until reaching the Promised Land.

The story is a genuine classic with as much drama as that of any modern adventure. Not only does it describe the trials and tribulations of Moses and the Hebrews, but it illustrates the many weaknesses of human character that surface under conditions of stress. The book is full of heavenly miracles from the plagues to the dramatic parting of the Red Sea. The story holds such fascination for us that we continually attempt to provide rational explanations for all these miracles.

A subject of great interest has always been manna, the food that God provided to the Hebrews during their forty-year sojourn in the desert. Manna appeared during the night as small grains covering the ground like frost. It appeared for the first time a little over a month after the Hebrews left Egypt and served as God's answer to their complaints of the difficulties of surviving desert life. Manna was not the only food available to the wandering Hebrews, since their goats furnished them with milk and cheese, and they were likely able to trade for flour and oil with other nomadic tribes traveling in the Sinai. But manna was the staple in their diet.

Because their diet was rather restricted, it was not long before the wandering Israelites began to complain bitterly about it. In his book *The Antiquities of the Jews*, Flavius Josephus, the famous Jewish historian, recounts what happened next:

> Having removed from the neighborhood of Mount Sinai, the Hebrews traveled from place to place, till they at length formed their encampment at Iseremoth (in the Sinai wilderness), where the multitude engaged in a sedition against Moses, telling him, that through his persuasions they had been seduced to abandon one of the most fertile parts of the whole world (Egypt), and now, instead of enjoying the blessings he had promised them they were obliged to wander from place to place in the utmost distress imaginable, being already on the point of perishing through the want of water; and they added, that if their manna should fail them they must inevitably fall victims to the miseries of famine.[6]

Talk about ingratitude! Here they were, rescued from a life of cruel and bitter slavery under harsh Egyptian taskmasters, and after a short interlude of freedom, they start to complain about their food. When they were reminded to be grateful for their liberty, they only complained more.

> He assured them that they should speedily have a supply of food sufficient for the maintenance of several days. However, they gave no credit to his promises, but violently exclaimed against him, one of them asking in scorn, by what means he could suppose himself capable of supplying so many thousand people with provisions? Hereupon he replied that notwithstanding their ingratitude they would be presently convinced that God and his servant Moses were still attentive to their welfare. Scarcely had he spoken these words, when an immense flight of quails descended into the camp, and the people gathered as many of them as they had occasion for.
>
> However, in a short time the Hebrews were severely punished

for their ingratitude and insolence; for the Almighty was pleased to afflict them with a plague, whereby great numbers of them were carried off. The place where they were visited with this terrible judgment is called Cabrothaba, or the graves of lust.

While eminently readable, the account of Flavius Josephus doesn't really tell us that much. He makes it clear that after complaining bitterly, the unappreciative Israelites suddenly appear to be blessed with an entire flock of quail to eat, but he goes on to describe how they were immediately afflicted with a terrible and fatal plague. Although he gives the circumstances and location (Cabrothaba) of this frightening event, Josephus provides few other clues that explain what actually happened. Fortunately, key details were carefully recorded in the original biblical record. Chapter 11 of the book of Numbers and verses 78 and 106 of the book of Psalms give a more complete and fearsome picture of what actually occurred.

While reading the account, it is worthwhile to try to imagine the scene—a people exhausted from travel and tired of eating the same old food day after day. Instead of rejoicing at the miracles that brought about their freedom, they complain that life had been better and more secure under the Egyptians. Upon witnessing this lack of appreciation for their newfound freedom and their incessant craving for meat in their diet, the Master of the Universe dramatically demonstrates his displeasure at this offensive behavior. The language used and the emotions described paint a frightening picture. I have highlighted some of the more significant passages in bold and made an observation (👁) here and there:

From the book of Numbers:

11:4. The mixed multitude among (the Israelites) began to have strong cravings, and the Israelites once again began to weep. "Who's going to give us some meat to eat?" they demanded.

11:5. "We fondly remember the fish that we could eat in Egypt at no cost, along with the cucumbers, melons, leeks, onions and garlic."

11:6. "But now **our spirits are dried up, with nothing but the manna** before our eyes."

11:10. Moses heard the people weeping with their families near the entrances of their tents. God became very angry, and Moses (also) considered it wrong.[7]

I find the next few verses quite disturbing. Just look at the language used to project God's anger. God is incensed with their ingratitude and also infuriated with their desire for meat, a primitive animal craving. God promises to punish that animal passion by providing the Israelites with so much meat that it will come out of their noses! It's pretty harsh material.

11:18. "Tell the people as follows: You have been whining in God's ears, saying, 'Who's going to give us some meat to eat? It was better for us in Egypt!' Now God is going to give you meat, and you will have to eat it."

11:19. "You will eat it not for one day, not for two days, not for five days, not for ten days, and not for twenty days."

11:20. "But for a full month (you will eat it) until it is coming out of your nose and making you nauseated. This is because you rejected God and you whined before Him, 'Why did we ever leave Egypt?'"

Finally, we come to the incident with the quails.

11:31. God caused a wind to start blowing, sweeping quail up from the sea. They ran out of strength over the camp, and (were flying) only two cubits above the ground for the distance of a day's journey in each direction.

11:32. The people went about all that day, all night, and the entire next day, and gathered quail. Even those who got the least had gathered ten chomers. [☞ A chomer is a little over six bushels.]

11:33. The meat was still between their teeth when (the people) began to die. God's anger was displayed against the people, and He struck them with an extremely severe plague. [👁 This is the first real clue—the meat was still between their teeth when they began to die.]

11:34. (Moses) named the place "Graves of Craving" (Kivroth HaTaavah), since it was in that place where they buried the people who had these cravings. [👁 Kivroth HaTaavah is the same as the Cabrothaba described in Josephus.]

This frightening story is repeated in Psalm 78:

78:27. He rained flesh also upon them as dust, and feathered fowls like as the sand of the sea:

78:28. And he let it fall in the midst of their camp, round about their habitations.

78:29. So they did eat, and were well filled: **for he gave them their own desire;**

78:30. They were not estranged from their lust. But while their meat was yet in their mouths,

78:31. The wrath of God came upon them, and **slew the fattest of them**, and smote down the chosen men of Israel.[8]

and again in Psalm 106:

106:14. But they had a **wanton craving** in the wilderness, and put God to the test in the desert;

106:15. He gave them what they asked, but sent a **wasting disease** among them.

What a series of events! The story portrays the Israelites' constant preoccupation with their physical rather than spiritual needs. At the heart of the issue is the human lusting for meat. It is their passion to submit to their animal desires that angers God. A miracle is created in order to bring the Israelites the meat they so gluttonously crave, but after they greedily set upon the quails to eat them, they begin to die immediately—*while the meat was still between their teeth!* Immediate retribution! What actually happened? Was it a mass food poisoning?

If we accept the description as accurate, this could not have been a foodborne infection like our modern *E. coli* O157:H7 or salmonella poisoning. Pathogenic foodborne bacteria take anywhere from eight to

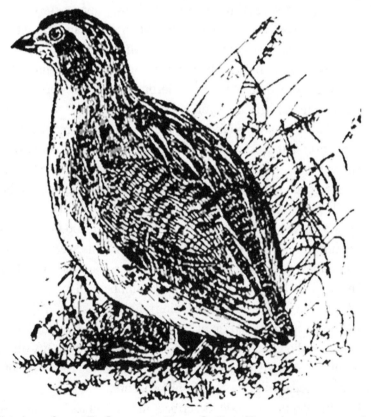

Quail taken from E. Sergent, "Les Cailles Empoisonneuses dans la Bible,—et en Alégrie de nos Jours," *Archives de l'Institute Pasteur d'Algérie* 19, no. 2 (1941): 161–92.

twenty-four hours or more to develop an infection sufficient for symptoms to be noticed. In this case, however, death occurred while the meat was still between the people's teeth—during or immediately after eating. There was no time for any type of infection to develop. The only thing that can make people ill that quickly is a foodborne toxin. How could quails flying in from the sea contain enough toxins to kill people immediately?

Quail hunting has been a common practice in the Mediterranean region from time immemorial. The European migratory quail (*Coturnix coturnix*) is found in Europe, Africa, and as far east as Pakistan and India. These little birds carry out a migratory flight twice every year. From August to October, as winter approaches, the birds leave Europe and fly south across the Mediterranean Sea and North Africa, all the way to equatorial Africa. After they fatten up over the winter, they begin to migrate back northward from late winter through early spring. The quail breed in Europe from late spring through summer and then begin the cycle all over again.

Not all the European quail follow the same migration route, however. Some fly over the western end of the Mediterranean, some over the middle, and some over the far eastern end. It is one of the easterly routes that we are concerned with, since this is the region described in the biblical quail episode. Starting out from eastern Europe, the quail fly through Greece and Turkey and then take the exhausting nonstop flight across the Mediterranean region to Egypt and Sinai. They continue along the Nile basin until they reach their final destination in equatorial East Africa.

The ancient Egyptians caught large numbers of quail when they landed after having crossed the Mediterranean. Fishermen spread their nets out on the ground and quickly trapped them as they landed on the shore, before the exhausted birds had an opportunity to lift off again. This tradition, carried out for millennia, still goes on today, despite the fact that the occasional food poisoning occurs.

The frightening episode described in the Bible has interested a number of medical and anthropology experts for many years. The first intensive study of the matter was carried out by Dr. Edmond Sergent, director of the Pasteur Institute in Algeria. In 1941, while war plans were being developed by Winston Churchill and Franklin Roosevelt to invade North Africa in order to deny the oil-rich Middle East to the German forces, Dr. Sergent, already world renowned for his work on malaria, published his initial studies on the poisonous quails of the Bible.[9]

Dr. Sergent had been intrigued by a publication he had recently come across. In his book *Yesterday and Today in Sinai*, Major C. S. Jarvis, former British governor of Sinai, described an incident of gastritis he had seen resulting from the consumption of quail in Sinai: ". . . and was no doubt the autumn migration when the birds arrive in clouds and are incidentally extraordinarily fat, which would account for the distressing outbreak of acute gastritis from which apparently the host suffered."[10] After Sergent read this account, he felt that the "acute gastritis" could only be the result of some form of intoxication rather than the "fat" that Jarvis referred to.

Sergent sent a letter outlining his idea of toxic quail to Major Jarvis, who quickly responded:

> You have raised quite a new point and the most interesting one. Although I have lived in Sinai for 14 years and have seen the two migrations of quails annually I have never heard of this "cailles toxiques" [toxic quails] but it is quite possible that this occurs only in Algeria. Of course on the spring migration the quails are returning from Central Africa and also they travel back quite slowly. For instance, in the Nile Valley some of them alight as far south as the Sudan border and work their way slowly northwards. They have the opportunity to eat of poisonous weeds on their way up. When they come south in the autumn, they fly straight from the cornfields of Hungary, Rumania and Russia and are in very good condition to eat.

Sergent went on to list the many references to poisonous quails written since the time of the Bible, including those of Lucretius, Didymus, and Pliny the Elder. He also made reference to the most famous physicians of ancient Islam, Avicenna and Ad-Damiri, who wrote that the quails fed on *Aconitum napellus* (wolfbane) and *Aconitum ferox* (ativisha), two extremely poisonous plants. Sergent made further reference to the publication of the French scientist Cornavin, who confirmed that quails were insensitive to the toxicity of the deadly plant *Conium maculatum* (hemlock) to a point where their bodies could contain enough toxins to kill the predators that eat them.[11]

Using the considerable facilities of the Pasteur Institute, Sergent carried out several experiments to determine the effect of feeding quails with hemlock seeds. He observed that the birds did not suffer from the paralysis that was so typical of hemlock poisoning. He then fed the same quail to dogs who immediately exhibited hind leg paralysis, the classic symptom of hemlock poisoning. In Sergent's mind, this experiment categorically solved the mystery of how the Israelites had died from consuming the quails.

Since the time of its original publication, Sergent's work was questioned by several other scientists and physicians. Some say the work was not conclusive and may have been technically flawed. They feel that other toxic plants or insects consumed by the quails were responsible for making the birds poisonous. Based on recent studies carried out in Greece and the Mediterranean islands, others felt that the ancient Israelites may possibly have had a genetic predisposition that made them particularly sensitive to some other type of quail toxin.[12] The most comprehensive review of the subject was made by Professor Louis Grivetti of the University of California, who highlighted in detail some of the contradictions between the biblical record and the hypotheses put forth by various scientists.[13]

Regardless of the type of toxin involved or the genetic predisposition of the Israelites, none of the scientists dispute that the story in the Bible is a vivid description of a mass food-poisoning incident. The exact direction of the wind from the sea and the present-day location where the incident took place are often speculated upon, but the phenomenon itself—the sudden abundance of quail presented to the Israelites—is never questioned.

Another view was given by Dr. Fred Rosner in his letters to the *Journal of the American Medical Association* in 1970 and again in 1978 to the *New England Journal of Medicine*: "An alternate explanation to the quail affair is that the entire happening was an act of God. . . . It is conceivable to attribute the deaths to both divine intervention as well as organic food poisoning if we interpret that God punished the people by medical means."[14] Thus we have the first record of mass food poisoning appearing in the Bible, a frightening episode intended to demonstrate God's retribution to those Israelites who submitted to the craving for meat. Lest we feel dissatisfied that scientists have not yet agreed upon the exact nature of the toxic agent involved in this biblical incident, it should be borne in mind that smaller outbreaks of quail poisoning continue to occur in the Mediterranean region to this day, but a definitive diagnosis of the responsible toxin has yet to be made.

EVENT 2. MY ASCLEPIUS IS DRAGON

In a subsequent section of the book of Numbers, there is yet another incident that begs explanation. It is not an example of a foodborne disease, but comes rather close—it is an example of a waterborne illness.

At a later time during their long sojourn in the wilderness, the Israelites find yet another excuse to complain against Moses and God, as recounted in chapter 21 of the book of Numbers.

> **21:5.** And the people spake against God, and against Moses, Wherefore have ye brought us up out of Egypt to die in the wilderness? For there is no bread, neither is there any water; and our soul loatheth this light bread.

> **21:6.** And the LORD sent fiery serpents among the people, and they bit the people; and much people of Israel died.

> **21:7.** Therefore the people came to Moses, and said, We have sinned, for we have spoken against the LORD, and against thee; pray unto the LORD, that he take away the serpents from us. And Moses prayed for the people.

21:8. And the LORD said unto Moses, Make thee a fiery serpent, and set it upon a pole: and it shall come to pass, that every one that is bitten, when he looketh upon it, shall live.

21:9. And Moses made a serpent of brass, and put it upon a pole, and it came to pass, that if a serpent had bitten any man, when he beheld the serpent of brass, he lived.[15]

This story is unique not only because it describes the disease but the cure as well. What were the fiery serpents and how could a brass representation of a serpent on a pole manage to cure this dreadful affliction?

In the eighteenth century, the famous Swedish naturalist Carolus Linnaeus (the father of modern biological taxonomy), first suggested that the "fiery serpents" mentioned in the Bible may have actually been parasitic worms common to the Middle East. This made sense because large worms were often described as serpents and a fiery serpent would be one that caused burning pain and discomfort.

A particularly nasty example of just such a parasitic worm common to the region described in the Bible is appropriately named *Dracunculus medinensis*, Dragon of Medina, and more commonly known today as the guinea worm. A female of the species can measure from three to eight feet in length but is less than an eighth of an inch in diameter. Males are only an inch or so in length. People become infected with these worms by drinking water containing minute copepods, called cyclops or water fleas, which have consumed the *Dracunculus* larvae.

When someone drinks contaminated water from shallow open wells or ponds, the cyclops become dissolved by the stomach acids and the hardy *Dracunculus* larvae are released and migrate through the intestinal wall. After maturing for about three months, males and females meet and quickly mate. The males eventually die in the tissues while the females continue to migrate along the major muscles. A year or so after the infection began, the pregnant females migrate to the surface of the skin where they cause painful blistering.

People infected with *Dracunculus* experience great pain and often

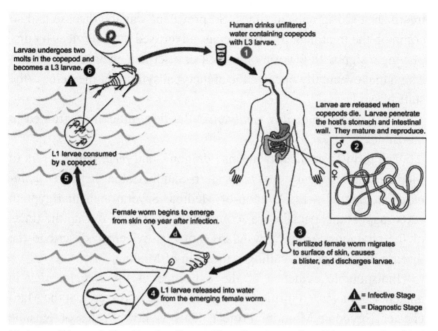

Guinea Worm Life Cycle, from the Centers for Disease Control and Prevention

try to relieve the burning sensation by soaking the infected part of their body in a pond or river. This stimulates the females to emerge and expel hundreds of thousands of larvae into the water, where they are greedily consumed by the voracious cyclops. Thus the cycle is repeated when people drink from the same source of water. The accompanying diagram shows the *Dracunculus* life cycle.[16]

This disease continues to exist in many parts of the tropical world (mainly Africa), and there still is no cure. If you visit the Web site of the US Centers for Disease Control and Prevention, you will find the following treatment prescribed: "Once the worm emerges from the wound, it can only be pulled out a few centimeters each day and wrapped around a small stick. Sometimes the worm can be pulled out completely within a few days, but this process usually takes weeks or months."[17]

In this day and age, such a treatment seems incredibly archaic, but that is all that can be done. In fact, this treatment is identical to the treatment used in ancient times. So prevalent was the disease and so common the treatment that physicians advertised their services by displaying a sign with a worm on a stick or a serpent encircling a staff— a sign that eventually became the archetypal symbol of medicine—the staff of Asclepius.

But was *Dracunculus medinensis* the fiery dragon mentioned in the Bible?

The term *Dracunculus* means "dragon," and *medinensis* refers to Medina, the legendary city in western Saudi Arabia, hence *Dracunculus medinensis*—the Dragon of Medina. Several ancient Egyptian texts suggest this parasite was common in the region during the times of the pharaohs. Arabic physicians, notably Avicenna, described the disease in great detail, calling it the Vein of Medina.

Indisputable evidence of the existence of the *Dracunculus* in ancient Egypt was confirmed during the course of research at the Manchester Egyptian Mummy Project. This is how Professor Rosalie David, who directed the Mummy Research Project at the Manchester Museum, answered the following interview question:

Speaking of disease, what do you consider the most interesting pathology found in the mummies to date?

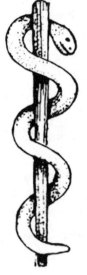

Perhaps the most interesting pathology we have found was in mummy No. 1770, which we autopsied in 1975. We found evidence of Guinea worm infestation—radiography revealed the calcified remains of a male Guinea worm in her abdominal wall. Her lower legs had been amputated probably about two weeks before death, possibly because they were ulcerated as the result of trying unsuccessfully to extract the female Guinea worms which sometimes try to break out and emerge through the skin on the legs.[18]

Staff of Asclepius, drawing by Mortin Satin.

This explanation supports the drinking of water infected with *Dracunculus medinensis* as a valid explanation for the fiery serpents mentioned in the Bible. In the book of Numbers, chapter 21, verse 5, the Israelites complained of no food and particularly of no water. With limited water resources for drinking or bathing, infection from guinea worms, which are endemic to the region, could very easily occur. Verse 6 describes fiery serpents and the typical symptoms of the painful *Dracunculus medinensis*. Incredibly, verses 8 and 9 describe the curing of the disease by setting the serpent upon a pole—the very same cure recommended today by the CDC, the world's most advanced center for disease control, and the cure that originated the symbol of the staff of Asclepius—the icon of modern medicine.

NOTES

1. N. de G. Davies and A. H. Gardiner, "The Tomb of Antifoker," Egypt Exploration Society (London: George Allen and Unwin, 1920).

2. World ORT, 2000, http://www.bible.ort.org/books/pentd2.asp?ACTION=displaypage&BOOK=1&CHAPTER=2 (accessed July 28, 2005).

3. Ibid., http://www.bible.ort.org/books/pentd2.asp?ACTION=displaypage&BOOK=1&CHAPTER=1 (accessed July 28, 2005).

4. Ibid., http://www.bible.ort.org/books/pentd2.asp?ACTION=displaypage&BOOK=1&CHAPTER=6 (accessed July 28, 2005).

5. Ibid., http://www.bible.ort.org/books/pentd2.asp?ACTION=displaypage&BOOK=1&CHAPTER=9 (accessed July 28, 2005).

6. C. Clarke, *The Whole Works of Flavius Josephus*, translated from the original Greek (Manchester: S. Russell, Deansgate, 1808).

7. World ORT, 2000, http://www.bible.ort.org/books/pentd2.asp?ACTION=displaypage&BOOK=4&CHAPTER=11 (accessed July 28, 2005).

8. Barnabas Ministries, BibleStudy.org, 2005, http://www.biblestudy.org/bibleref/av/ps078.html (accessed July 28, 2005).

9. E. Sergent, "Les Cailles Empoisonneuses Dans La Bible,—et en Algérie de nos Jours," *Archives de L'Institute Pasteur D'Algérie* 19, no. 2 (1941): 161–92.

10. C. S. Jarvis, *Yesterday and Today in Sinai* (London: Blackwood and Sons, 1931).

11. C. Cornavin, *Des Plantes Vénéneuses et des Empoisonnements qu'elles Déterminant* (Paris: Firmin-Didot, 1887).

12. T. Ouzounellis, "Some Notes on Quail Poisoning," *Journal of the American Medical Association* 211, no. 7 (1970): 1186.

13. L. Grivetti, "Reading 13: Coturnism (Part 1)," Nutrition 120A., Nutrition Department, University of California, Davis, 2002, http://64.233 .179.104/search?q=cache:wOj9sQy6SzIJ:teaching.ucdavis.edu/nut120a/004 1.htm+louis+grivetti+quail&hl=en (accessed July 28, 2005) and "Reading 13: Coturnism (Part 2)," http://64.233.179.104/search?q=cache:fJ3H_zU1 adwJ:teaching.ucdavis.edu/nut120a/0042.htm+louis+grivetti+quail&hl=en (accessed July 28, 2005).

14. F. Rosner, "Biblical Quail Incident," *Journal of the American Medical Association* 211, no. 9 (1970): 1544; F. Rosner, "Biblical Quail Incident," *New England Journal of Medicine* 298, no. 1 (1978): 57.

15. The Bible, Web Book Publications, 2005, http://www.web-books .com/Classics/Bible/Numbers/Numbers21.htm (accessed July 28, 2005).

16. The Board of Trustees of the University of South Carolina, Microbiology and Immunology, 2004, http://pathmicro.med.sc.edu/parasitology/ Dracunculiasis-lc.gif (accessed July 28, 2005).

17. "What Is the Treatment for Guinea Worm Disease?" Centers for Disease Control and Prevention, Atlanta, GA, http://www.cdc.gov/ncidod/ dpd/parasites/dracunculiasis/factsht_dracunculiasis.htm#treatment (accessed July 28, 2005).

18. R. David, "Speaking of Disease, What Do You Consider the Most Interesting Pathology Found in the Mummies to Date?" http://www .archaeology.org/online/features/mummies/ (accessed July 28, 2005).

CHAPTER 2
THE GREEKS AND ROMANS
(1200 BCE–500 CE)

The Greek and Roman dedication to science and philosophy resulted in an explosion of practical technology to improve agriculture and food processing. Although these developments made foods and beverages tastier and more acceptable, it did not necessarily result in greater food safety. On the contrary, as we shall see, some developments resulted in an orgy of poisoning that endured for more than two thousand years.

The Greeks and Romans not only enjoyed a splendid Mediterranean diet but also shared similar eating habits. Most sources agree that they generally ate three meals a day, although the very poor were happy to enjoy a single daily meal.

Breakfast consisted of bread, olives, cheese, and olive oil. Lunch would likely be made up of bread, cheese, and some fruit. Dinner was the main meal of the day and consisted of vegetables and olive oil for the lower classes or a more elaborate multicourse meal for the wealthy. In such a meal, the first appetizer course would contain salads, eggs, mushrooms, or shellfish. The second course might have poultry, pork, game, or fish—all served with various vegetables. The final course would offer fruits and sweets and, as with all other courses, wine.

The great expanse of the Roman Empire allowed it to import a wide variety of foods, spices, and herbs, giving its population a taste for exotic dishes with highly flavored and spicy sauces. This bounty contributed to the custom of eating and drinking to excess—the most popular of habits to be exported throughout the domain.

The Romans were experts in aquaculture. If you visit the Italian coastline between Rome and Naples today, you will see evidence of the ancient Roman aquaculture ponds in which a great variety of fish and eels were produced for the table. At the famous Grotto of Tiberius, which is located at the south end of my favorite beach, Sperlonga, there is a very large aquaculture pond that incorporates a small island where ancient Roman diners would eat and enjoy the antics of the fish swimming and feeding all around them.

The style of consumption also designated social boundaries. As an example, men and women ate and drank different foods and beverages, while priests and other religious officials followed their own strict dietary regimes. The most obvious difference was between the affluent and the poor, with the rich exhibiting their wealth through the most extravagant banquets. This is occasionally mimicked today by those with more money than propriety.

Food was instrumental in projecting the glory that was Greece and the grandeur that was Rome. But it also contributed to their downfall. It was the Greek and Roman bacchanalian love of food and particularly drink that served as the origin of the world's longest bout of chronic poisoning—one that plagued the Western world for two millennia.

EVENT 3. THE GORY THAT WAS GREECE

The Golden Age of Greece was brought short by Sparta—the most powerful state of Peloponnesus—which attacked Athens in 431 BCE, beginning the brutal twenty-seven-year-long Peloponnesian War. The casualties were enormous, with one out of every four Athenians dying very soon after the war began. These casualties were not caused by battle, however, but rather by a terrible plague, which spread throughout the city.

Sparta blockaded the walls of the city, preventing the people of Athens from getting supplies of fresh food from the countryside. Faced with famine, starvation, and so many casualties, Athens finally surrendered to Sparta in 404 BCE. Thus, one of the greatest periods of classical human enlightenment passed ignominiously into history.

Because the Plague of Athens played such a critical role in the outcome of the Peloponnesian War, the subject has occupied scholars for many years. What caused the plague? Various theories have suggested that it could have been caused by bubonic plague, dengue fever, Ebola virus, influenza, or measles, but each of these is unlikely because the symptoms described in the comprehensive historical record written by Thucydides do not match those diseases. More recently, it has been suggested that the Plague of Athens was an epidemic of typhus fever, because it hit hardest during times of war and both have similar mortality rates. To further support this theory, reference has been made to a striking complication of the plague: gangrene of the tips of the fingers and toes. However, this clue supports a far more logical explanation that involves the consumption of contaminated food.

We are fortunate to have an eyewitness account of the events from Thucydides, who lived in Athens during the plague and wrote *The History of the Peloponnesian War* in 431 BCE. His description of the plague and a detailed description of the symptoms of the victims can be found in chapter 7, *Second Year of the War—The Plague of Athens*, translated by Richard Crawley:

> ... people in good health were all of a sudden attacked by violent heats in the head, and redness and inflammation in the eyes, the inward parts, such as the throat or tongue. ... When it fixed in the stomach, it upset it; and discharges of bile of every kind named by physicians ensued, accompanied by very great distress. ... Externally the body was not very hot to the touch, nor pale in its appearance, but reddish, livid, and breaking out into small pustules and ulcers. But internally it burned so that the patient could not bear to

have on him clothing or linen even of the very lightest description. ...What they would have liked best would have been to throw themselves into cold water; as indeed was done by some of the neglected sick, who plunged into the rain-tanks in their agonies of unquenchable thirst; though it made no difference whether they drank little or much . . . when they succumbed, as in most cases, on the seventh or eighth day to the internal inflammation, they had still some strength in them . . . even where it did not prove mortal, it still left its mark on the extremities; the fingers and the toes, and many escaped with the loss of these, some too with that of their eyes.[1]

All in all, it was pretty miserable stuff that challenges the description of most of the diseases that have been suggested. Yet, more than a century ago, Rudolf Kobert suggested that the Athenians may have been experiencing ergotism—the long-term effect of ergot poisoning.[2] This idea was immediately challenged, because ergot is found mainly on rye, a grain the Athenians did not traditionally eat. However, the Athenians did eat wheat and a very similar disease resulting from moldy wheat is called Alimentary Toxic Aleukia or ATA.

From the account of Thucydides, it is clear that the disease abnormally affected the upper classes out of all proportion to the other citizens of Athens. In fact, only the upper classes could afford to eat wheat. The Greek historian Diodorus Siculus mentions that the grain the Athenians were eating at that time was bad, most likely the result of poor storage conditions. In wheat, these conditions encourage the growth of the *Fusarium* mold, which produces the virulent T-2 toxin responsible for ATA.

ATA symptoms follow four separate stages. In the first stage, the disease is hardly noticed. Some patients experience a burning sensation in the mouth and the gastrointestinal tract, and occasionally the

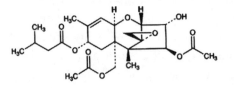

T-2 Toxin, molecular drawing prepared by Morton Satin.

tongue feels slightly swollen. After some days, the symptoms worsen and lead to vomiting, diarrhea, and generalized gastric pain. Body temperatures usually are normal, and, strangely, many people seem to experience a full recovery after this stage has run its course.

Unfortunately, the second stage of this disease follows two to four weeks later when the victim feels relatively well. During this period there is a growing breakdown of bone marrow and the eventual appearance of splotchy petechiae (little broken capillaries) on the body. At stage three, as a result of the massive bone marrow break-down, the victim has greatly decreased resistance and experiences larger hemorrhaging all over the skin and limbs. Small, inflamed pus-filled lesions on the surface of the skin often occur, followed by necrosis of the extremities, a condition clearly described by Thucy-dides. It is at this stage that death may occur.

Large areas of the former Soviet Union have been subject to out-breaks of ATA. Although first reported in the nineteenth century, the largest outbreaks occurred in the 1930s and again in the 1940s, during World War II. Upward of a quarter of a million people died of this dis-ease from 1942 to 1944.

The final stage of the disease is reserved for those who actually recover and is characterized by a gradual replenishment of bone marrow and an improvement in the white blood cell count. Full re-covery can occur, but over an extended period of time. Unfortunately, for the Athenians and the Golden Age of Greece, time had run out.

EVENT 4. BEWARE OF GREEKS BEARING HONEY

In his chronicle *The Anabasis*, the Greek historian and general Xenophon provided the Western world's first eyewitness account of a great military campaign. He describes how, in 401 BCE, a band of ten thousand undisciplined Greek mercenaries first traveled east to fight for Cyrus the Younger in the Persian prince's attempt to usurp the throne from his brother. The campaign ended in a disastrous retreat characterized by the murder, rape, robbery, and enslavement of countless innocent villagers in the lands through which the Greek mercenary army passed.

On their trek back to Greece, the disheartened soldiers looted whatever they could from the local inhabitants. This included food; honey in particular was high on the list of sought-after commodities. In the territory of Colchis, by the Black Sea, Xenophon's men raided the local supply of beehives. After gorging themselves on the honey, they became intoxicated and were seized with fits of vomiting and nausea. They became totally disoriented and ran about like madmen. Xenophon was very lucky because the pursuing Colchian army did not attack the men who were completely incapable of defending themselves. It took some days to recover, and the ragtag mercenaries moved westward as quickly as possible to get to more hospitable territory.

History so often repeats itself, and in 67 BCE, Rome, perceiving a threat to its territories, sent out the great General Pompey to conquer King Mithridates IV of Pontus. Over the course of several battles, Mithridates gradually retreated until his army was forced to face off with the Romans near the city of Trabzon on the Black Sea coast of Turkey. Pompey, who was certain that Mithridates' retreat was chaotic and illogical, was unaware that it had been carefully planned by the king's chief adviser.

Pompey's troops were in honey country, and it didn't take them long before they plundered the region's hives. In a carbon copy of the antics of Xenophon's army, Pompey's men gorged themselves on honeycombs and became intoxicated. This time Mithridates took advantage of the situation and massacred three squadrons of Pompey's troops while they were still under the influence of the honey's toxins.

Despite this setback, Rome eventually gained full control of the area around the Black Sea, but had never before come so close to a "sweet surrender."

It's hard for most people to believe that a food as historically significant and universally trusted as natural honey can, under certain circumstances, be quite toxic. However, that is the case, because when bees collect their nectar from rhododendrons or laurel, both members of the botanical family Ericaceae, they also bring along grayanotoxin, the poison these plants contain.

When the bees carry out their marvelous transformation of nectar to honey, they concentrate the level of grayanotoxin in the final product to a degree that it becomes toxic to consumers. Grayanotoxin binds to the sodium channels in cell membranes and prevents the inactivation of excitable nerve and muscle cells, which are then maintained in a state of depolarization. The central nervous system and the skeletal and heart muscles are in a highly agitated state, which causes the sort of madness described in the historical events.

Honey madness is not a condition restricted to the Mediterranean region. In the year 946, Prince Igor's widow, Olga, together with her son, took their revenge upon their enemies, the Derevlians. She sent word to the Derevlians that she was coming to mourn at her husband's grave. When she arrived at Prince Igor's tomb, she wept bitterly and bade her followers prepare a great funeral feast. When the Derevlians sat down to drink, they were offered mead made from mad honey. When the Derevlians were drunk, Olga and her followers massacred all five thousand of them. Sweet!

Mad honey was also found in the New World. The eastern half of North America has been recording episodes of honey intoxication for centuries. A review of honey poisoning in North America was first read to the American Philosophical Society as early as 1794, although it was not published until 1802.[3]

Shortly thereafter, Abraham Lincoln—destined to become the sixteenth president of the United States—was born. Among the many quotations attributed to him is one fitting to the role of honey in history: "When the conduct of men is designed to be influenced, persuasion, kind unassuming persuasion, should ever be adopted. It is an old and true maxim that a drop of honey catches more flies than a gallon of gall."

EVENT 5. GET THE LEAD OUT

Of the seven famous metals of antiquity (gold, copper, silver, lead, tin, iron, and mercury), the ready availability of lead and the ease of casting it into useful products made its use extremely widespread. Lead is not normally found free in nature but is produced from the natural lead sulfide ore called galena. The mining of lead started around 6000 BCE. A necklace from that age made of smelted lead was found in Anatolia, Turkey. Galena was first used by the ancient Egyptians to make ornaments or eye paint. Metallic lead is easily produced from galena simply by heating it in a camp fire. By 3500 BCE, lead was used widely as a material for containers and pipes. Ancient pipes with the insignia of the Roman emperors can still be found. The chemical symbol for lead is Pb, from the Latin word *plumbum*, which also happens to be the root of the word for the tradesmen who worked with pipes—plumbers.

Many historians believe that it was the lead pipes carrying the water supply that led to the downfall of the Roman Empire. While there is no doubt that lead pipes slightly increased the risk of lead poisoning, the pipes represented a relatively minor hazard to health. Both the Greeks and the Romans discovered a more insidious application of lead that exposed them to a far greater risk.

They found that when they coated the interiors of their copper or bronze cooking pots with lead, most of the food and beverages they prepared tasted much better. Nowhere was this more evident than in the preparation of acidic products such as wines. Popular recipes of the day called for the boiling of grape must (juice pressed from grapes before it has fermented) in lead-lined vessels in order to prepare a liquid additive that would enhance the color, flavor, and shelf life of wine. The grape must was boiled until it was reduced by half in volume. The resultant thick, syrupy liquid was called *sapa*—a term for concentrated grape juice still used in Italian cooking.

What actually happened when the must was boiled in lead vessels was a reaction between the acetic acid from the grape ferment and the

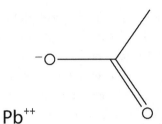

Lead acetate, molecular drawing prepared by Morton Satin.

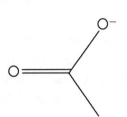

lead of the pot to form a compound called lead acetate. Lead acetate is also called lead sugar because it is so sweet. This compound added just the right type of sweetness to bring out the best in wines and corrected many of the souring problems winemakers routinely encountered. The problem was that sapa prepared using the ancient formulas contained between a quarter and one gram of lead per liter! A single teaspoon of liquid sapa was more than enough to cause lead poisoning, but no one understood this at the time. In fact, because its effects were long term rather than immediate, the relationship between lead and disease was not well understood for another two thousand years.

Hippocrates (460–377 BCE) was the first physician to link the excess consumption of food and wine with lead-based gout. The first undisputed account of lead poisoning was written in the second century BCE by Nicander of Colophon (197–130 BCE), a renowned botanist and physician. He described symptoms of intense intestinal pains and tissue swelling. Several other ancient notables such as Pliny the Elder (23–79 CE) and Dioscorides (40–90 CE) specifically warned that the consumption of wine, particularly sapa-corrected wine, would result in severe nervous disorders—but to no avail. The practice of consuming wine laced with lead sugar continued unabated and was exacerbated by the consumption of several other foods that were sweetened with sapa.

This constant ingestion of lead by large segments of the population resulted in a series of epidemics throughout the Roman Empire. The average consumption of wine per person was estimated to be more than a liter a day. Little wonder that so many well-known Romans were considered to be dim-witted. Emperor Claudius limped, slurred his words, had fits and tremors, and slobbered. Since he was a known glutton and heavy drinker, it seems likely that many of his symptoms were the result of lead poisoning. Many Roman emperors were thought to be heavy drinkers and mentally disturbed enough to be considered today as prime candidates for lead poisoning. One publication goes so far as to suggest that more than two-thirds of the leading Roman aristocrats, who served between 30 and 220 CE, were most likely victims of lead poisoning.[4] The disease became endemic throughout most of Europe, particularly among the wealthy, who could afford to consume a good deal of wine that had been sweetened with sapa. When a rib bone of Pope Clement (who died in 1047) was analyzed, it revealed enough lead to support the conclusion that he had died of chronic lead poisoning.[5]

During the course of these epidemics, chroniclers wrote of painful stomach colic, epilepsy, and paralysis as typical symptoms. The disease variously became known as the *huttenkatz* of Germany (the "cat of the foundries," because it tore at the entrails like a cat) and the colic of Devonshire; however, the most common term used in the medical literature from the seventeenth century onward was the colic of Poitou. The term was first coined in 1639 by François Citois, the personal physician of Cardinal Richelieu. He was describing a disease that started in the region of Poitou in western France in the year 1572 and continued unabated for almost seventy years. Like many physicians of his time, he attributed the disease to God's wrath upon the sinful people. Here are the rather graphic terms Citois used to describe the symptoms:

A new colic disease named "bilious" for the most bitter pains from the bile has arisen and is even now spreading . . . the bodies' extremities are cold, strength languishes, the spirit is disturbed, the body restless, sleeplessness is continuous, there is lethargy and frequent chest pains, loss of appetite, constant nausea, belching, vomiting; . . . burning pain in the epigastrium sometimes . . . very sharp pain in the stomach, intestines, loins and groin racks the patient . . . ; Soon, as the poison spreads, the upper arms, breasts and whole chest feels as though plucked, pricked and pierced by needles.[6]

It is not difficult to understand the mechanism and course of the disease. Lead ions are attracted and bound to the natural sulfhydryl groups that are common to most of our proteins. In the case of enzyme proteins, this binding interferes with their normal action and results in a wide range of symptoms, the most important being the negative effects on the nervous system. Paralysis develops slowly, with the greatest pain resulting from the inaction of the intestine, which thereby causes cramps and constipation.

In the Imperial German city of Ulm at the head of the Danube, there were outbreaks of the colic of Poitou in two local monasteries in 1694. The attending physician was Dr. Eberhard Gockel, a very astute and practical physician. He noted that those monks who did not drink wine did not suffer from the colic, while those who did drink wine got sick. In fact, he tasted their wine often enough to develop a mild form of the colic himself.

In order to investigate the matter further, he spoke to a local manufacturer who showed him how the recent productions of wine were treated to overcome their sourness, which had resulted from a spell of poor weather for a number of years. Litharge, or lead oxide, was routinely added to the region's wines as a sweetening agent. Gockel went home and tried to duplicate this phenomenon. He was very successful and was able to instantly turn an undrinkable acidic wine into the best of products. He quickly deduced that the wine was the source of the colic problem and two years later published a medical paper describing the great harm that can befall anyone drinking "corrected" wines. He even developed a method to detect the presence of lead in wines.

Other physicians in the area confirmed Gockel's conclusions, and the whole matter came to the attention of Salomon Reisel, the personal physician of Duke Eberhard Ludwig. The duke quickly issued an edict forbidding the adulteration of wine with litharge on pain of death—not only for the adulterators but for anyone who knew of them but didn't turn them in. A few years later, Johanne Ehrni, a barrel maker from Eisslingen, was tried and convicted of the crime of adulterating wine with lead and publicly beheaded in Stuttgart![7]

Despite this incident, the relationship between adulterated wine and the colic of Poitou received little attention, and the practice continued unabated in other regions. As late as 1884, it was reported that wines from the Samur region of France were sweetened by adding lead pellets.[8]

In 1703, shortly after Gockel published his work on the colic of Poitou, a well-known British physician named Musgrave published a treatise on gout.[9] It was Musgrave's contention that attacks of gout were precipitated by the colic. He was particularly concerned with the colic of Devonshire, the region that was well known for the conspicuous consumption of a rough and acidic cider and the region wherein the colic was endemic. He stressed that in those years when the apple harvests were small and manageable, the colic never appeared. He went on to say that the colic was often followed with pains in the joints, swelling, and all the typical symptoms of gout. Because Musgrave's chief concern was the relationship between the Devonshire colic and gout, he did not take the theory one step further and relate it to the consumption of lead in the cider, even though his patients' symptoms were similar to those of the colic of Poitou.

A young colleague of Musgrave's by the name of John Huxham continued work on the Devonshire colic and published a long essay on the subject in 1739. The essay was in Latin, and it was twenty years before it was published in English. He described the severe outbreak that occurred in 1724 and provided a full account of the symptoms.

Huxham noticed that with some patients the symptoms might cease but would return again after drinking cider. Because that particular year was a bumper crop for apples, most of them went into the

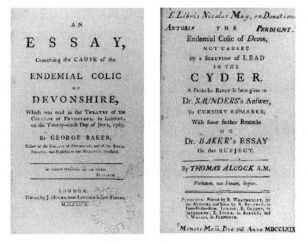

Left taken from R. S. M. McConaghy, "Sir George Baker and
the Devonshire Colic," *Medical History* 11, no. 4 (1967): 345–60.
Right taken from "Devon Colic," Wikipedia, http://en.wikipedia
.org/wiki/Devon_colic (accessed June 5, 2006).

production of cider. Cider was so cheap it became a major source of
calories for the poor. His theory was that the colic was due to the consumption of cider before it was properly fermented. Like Musgrave
before him, Huxham did not associate the Devonshire colic with the
colic of Poitou, and hence the relationship to the consumption of lead
was not made.

Nothing further was done to mitigate the devastating impact of the
Devonshire colic until 1767, when Sir George Baker, the eminent
court physician and himself a Devonian, published a pamphlet
warning his countrymen of the dangers of drinking the local cider. He
kindly gave credit to the publications of Musgrave and Huxham, but
went on to say that he believed they missed the mark in discerning the
cause of the disease. He stated that there was nothing wrong with pure
cider and that the cause of the colic was cider adulterated with lead.

Baker found out that a particular characteristic of the apple presses
in Devonshire was the use of lead sheeting as an inner lining to prevent leaking. In other counties such as Hereford, Gloucester, and

Worcester, the apple presses were very similar, except that there was no lead used in their construction. Further analytical experiments proved that cider from Devonshire was heavily contaminated with lead while those from the other counties were not.

A predictable storm of protest broke out in Devonshire. Farmers were concerned that Baker's essay would kill their cider business. A number of opposing essays were written refuting Baker's conclusions, some of which were very influential in reducing the immediate impact of his publication. The most credible criticism came from a Dr. James Hardy, who actually agreed with Baker that the colic was due to lead poisoning. However, he contended that the source of lead was not the apple presses but rather the lead-glazed pottery in which the cider was sold—a theory that gained little recognition at the time, although it has become accepted in modern times. Baker's opinion held out, and within a short period more modern mechanical presses without lead components began producing lead-free cider. The centuries-old endemic colic of Devonshire finally disappeared.

It is interesting to learn that Benjamin Franklin corresponded with Sir George Baker on the subject of lead poisoning. Franklin was interested in the subject, since he had served as a printer's apprentice. He had always linked the practice of cleaning lead type by the use of heating with a condition called Dangles—a permanent wrist drop that many older typesetters had. In 1745 he published a paper written by Dr. Thomas Cadwalader on the subject of dry gripes in the West Indies. Dry gripes were the intestinal pains common in cases of lead poisoning, and Cadwalader attributed the disease to the consumption of rum that had been distilled using certain equipment—where the still heads and worm condensers were made of lead or lead alloys such as pewter, which contained from 10 to 20 percent lead.

Franklin supported Baker's theory that the lead in cider was the causative factor in the Devonshire colic. Baker used the endorsement of so eminent a person to further prop up his case. In 1767, in the company of Sir John Pringle, a renowned British physician, Franklin visited La Charité Hospital in Paris. La Charité was famous for curing patients who had the Poitou colic symptoms. Franklin was a very observant person and noted that most of the patients worked in a trade in which lead was used. Almost twenty years later, on July 31, 1786, he wrote a long letter to his friend Benjamin Vaughan, confirming his belief that lead was the cause of the centuries-old epidemic of lead poisoning. He ended the letter with: "You will see by it, that the Opinion of the Mischievous effect from Lead is at least above Sixty Years old; and you will observe with Concern how long a useful Truth may be known, and exist, before it is generally reciev'd and practic'd on."[10]

Franklin's reference to "at least above Sixty years old" certainly predates the work of Baker and Cadwalader. It refers to the passage of an act in Massachusetts in 1723, which prohibited the distillation of rum and other strong liquors in stills where the still heads and condensers were made of lead or lead alloys.[11] This act was likely based on the relationship between the consumption of rum and the typical symptoms of lead poisoning as well as Gockel's publication on the colic of Poitou. As a result, many citizens of Massachusetts were spared the ravages of lead poisoning, while much of the rest of the rum-drinking world suffered from it.

It is interesting to note the archaeological evidence from a colonial plantation cemetery (1670–1730) in Virginia. There were two main groups buried there: the white plantation owners were in the north section while their slave laborers were in the south section. The bones of the northern group contained five times as much lead as those of the southern group, clearly demonstrating that lead ingestion was far greater among the wealthy.[12]

EVENT 6. WHEN IN DOUBT, ASSUME THE GOUT

Gout is a complex disease caused by faulty metabolism, which results in high levels of uric acid in the blood. People with gout have either an increased production of uric acid or an impaired excretion of uric acid,

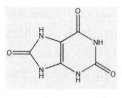

Uric acid, molecular drawing prepared by Morton Satin.

or a combination of both conditions. A diet rich in alcohol, wine, and high-protein foods, such as meat, has always been considered responsible for individual attacks.

Crystals of uric acid form inside the joints and cause intense pain whenever the area is moved or flexed. The inflammation of the tissues around the affected joint also causes the skin to swell and become extremely tender and sore to the slightest touch. Even a light dressing can be extremely painful on an affected joint. Attacks of gout can be agonizing and can cause an otherwise capable person to be totally dysfunctional.

Gout has been described in one form or another since the earliest

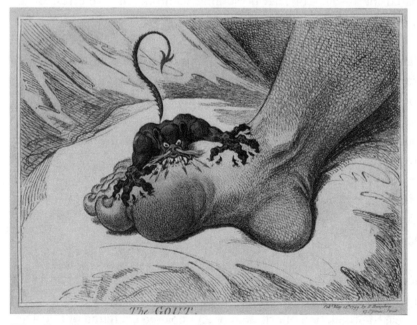

The Gout by James Gilray, 1799.

of Greek writings. Although it was always linked with the lifestyles of the rich and famous, it was never directly associated with lead poisoning.[13] The wealthy ate and drank the very best, so gout was attributed to the richness of their diet rather than anything else. It was called *Morbus Dominorum*—the disease of the gods. That explanation for gout continued to be accepted throughout the ages and is still the most common rationale for the disease today.

The predilection of gout for wealthy and powerful victims resulted in the disease's becoming the theme of humorous satire. This was understandable, since some of the most dreadful rulers of Europe from the fourteenth to the nineteenth centuries numbered among its many sufferers. The kings of France, the Bourbons of Spain, the Medicis, the Hapsburgs, and the Tudor, Stuart, and Hanover sovereigns of England all endured the ravages of this disease.

Unexpectedly, the number of gout sufferers in Britain increased dramatically when the tariffs on Portuguese wines were reduced (in accordance with the 1703 Treaty of Methuen), allowing these wines into the country at a lower price than French wines. George Frideric Handel, after moving to England to become court composer for Britain's royalty, drank considerable quantities of port as can be deduced from a penciled note in one of his manuscripts: "12 gallons port, 12 bottles French, Duke Street, Meels."[14] It is thus very possible that he suffered from gout induced by lead poisoning.[15]

Port wine is fortified with brandy that is added during the fermentation process. This stops the development of the wine while it is still sweet and fruity. Lead was a routine contaminant in the old Portuguese method of distilling brandy because the levels found in port products produced between 1770 and 1820 varied from 320 to 1,900 micrograms per liter![16]

When lead was finally considered to be a primary factor in the development of gout, the disease was called "saturnine gout" because in ancient alchemy, metals were always affiliated with specific planets, and lead's associate was Saturn. Lead is a strong contributory factor to gout because of its negative effect on the excretion of uric acid by the kidneys.

In one way or another, consumers have suffered from lead poisoning for more than two thousand years. Lead poisoning continues today with bootleg moonshine produced in the United States. When the fermented corn mash is distilled, it is occasionally condensed through old automobile radiators that have joints and patches made with old lead-based solder. The acidic alcohol vapor leaches the lead out of the solder and contaminates the moonshine. In a recent article describing a study performed in a large urban area where the patients admitted consuming moonshine during the previous five years, more than half had elevated levels of lead in their blood and a third had very elevated levels.[17]

Considering its disastrous impact upon people throughout the ages, we should all agree that it's time to get the lead out!

NOTES

1. Daniel C. Stevenson, *The History of the Peloponnesian War by Thucydides*, trans. Richard Crawley, Internet Classics Archive, 1994–2000, http://classics.mit.edu/Thucydides/pelopwar.html (accessed July 28, 2005).

2. R. Kobert, "Ueber die Pest des Thukydides," *Janus* 4 (1899): 244–99.

3. B. S. Barton, "Account of the Poisonous and Injurious Honey of North America," *Transactions of the American Philosophical Society* 5 (1802): 51–70.

4. J. O. Nriagu, "Saturnine Gout among Roman Aristocrats," *New England Journal of Medicine* 308, no. 11 (1983): 660–63.

5. W. Specht and K. Fischer, "Vergiftungsnachweis an den Resten einer 900 Jahre alten Leiche," *Archiv für Kriminologie* 124 (1959): 61–84.

6. F. Citois, "De Novo et populari apud Pictones dolore colico bilioso diatriba," *Opuscula Medica* (Paris: Sébastien Cramoisy, 1639).

7. J. Eisinger, "Lead and Wine—Eberhard Gockel and the Colica Pictonum," *Medical History* 26 (1982): 279–302.

8. K. B. Hofmann, "Das Blei bie den Völkern des Alterums," in *Beiträge aus der Geshichte der Chemie*, ed. F. Dentike (Leipzig and Vienna, 1885).

9. H. A. Waldron, "The Devonshire Colic," *Journal of the History of Medicine* 25, no. 4 (1970): 383–413.

10. Jean Spencer Felton, "Man, Medicine and Work in America: A Historical Series, III. Benjamin Franklin and His Awareness of Lead Poisoning," *Journal of Occupational Medicine* 9, no. 11 (1967): 543–54.

11. "An Act for Preventing Abuses in Distilling of Rum and Other Strong Liquors, with Leaden Heads or Pipes," *Massachusetts Acts and Resolves* (September 3, 1723).

12. A. C. Aufderheide et al., "Lead in Bone II: Skeletal-Lead Content as an Indicator of Lifetime Lead Ingestion and the Social Correlates in an Archeological Population," *American Journal of Physical Anthropology* 55 (1981): 285–91.

13. T. Appelboom and J. C. Bennett, "Gout of the Rich and Famous," *Journal of Rheumatology* 13, no. 3 (1986): 618–22.

14. A. Fuller-Maitland and A. H. Mann, *Catalogue of the Music in the Fitzwilliam Museum, Cambridge* (London: C. J. Clay and Sons, Cambridge University Press Warehouse, 1893), p. 194.

15. W. A. Frosch, "The Case of George Frideric Handel," *New England Journal of Medicine* 321, no. 11 (1989): 765–69.

16. G. V. Ball, "Two Epidemics of Gout," *Bulletin of the History of Medicine* 45, no. 5 (1971): 401–408.

17. B. W. Morgan, K. H. Todd, and B. Moore, "Elevated Blood Lead Levels in Urban Moonshine Drinkers," *Annals of Emergency Medicine* 37, no. 1 (2001): 51–54.

PART II
THE MIDDLE AGES

CHAPTER 3
THE MIDDLE AGES
(500–1500 CE)

The period of time between the fall of the Roman Empire and the middle of the fifteenth century is commonly referred to as the Middle Ages. The precise dates of the beginning and end of this period are fairly arbitrary, depending upon which particular events in history are stressed. As an example, the year 476 is often considered to be the beginning of the Middle Ages because that is when the last Roman emperor, Romulus Augustus, was deposed. Of course, the destruction of the Roman Empire did not take place on that one day but was the culmination of a century-long regression of Roman power throughout its empire. As a consequence, some consider the year 375 as the beginning of the Middle Ages because that is when the Huns first embarked on the systematic destruction of Rome's Western Empire.

The exact dates of the close of the Middle Ages are similarly under debate. Some historians link it to the rise of the Renaissance in Italy in the fourteenth century, while others link it to the fall of Constantinople or the discovery of America by Columbus, both of which occurred in the fifteenth century. What is important is that it was a period of dramatic population and cultural change.

The established society went through changes in law, culture, religion, and patterns of property ownership. The rule of Roman law (Pax Romana), with its guaranteed benefits of safe trade and manufacture and the promise of a better life for many of its citizens, drew to a close. It was replaced by the rule of local warlords and kings, resulting in a dramatic change in the economic and social norms as well as a general degradation of the physical infrastructure. This in turn rapidly evolved into a feudal system wherein the overlord (usually a king) awarded land grants, or fiefs, to his most important cronies and the prelates of his church. At the bottom of society's ladder were the peasants or serfs who worked the lord's land in exchange for his protection.

EVENT 7. THERE'S FUNGUS AMONG US

**There may be old mushroom hunters,
and there may be bold mushroom hunters,
but there are no old and bold mushroom hunters!**

Humans have been blessed and cursed with fungi from the dawn of civilization. These organisms are neither plant nor animal but maintain some characteristics of each. Fungi can't move about like an animal nor do they have chlorophyll like plants. They don't produce their own energy, but they must consume organic matter to survive. Unlike the primitive prokaryote bacteria, fungal cells have a true nucleus and can sexually reproduce. However, fungi can also reproduce through the employment of spores similar to some of the more primitive plants such as ferns and mosses. Although reproduction takes place in both manners, modern studies indicate that fungi are more closely related to animals than to plants.

Most fungi are made up of delicate hairlike tubes called hyphae, which reproduce by elongation and branching. A mass of hyphae is called mycelium—a structure that can be formed into anything from the furry mold you see growing on the strawberries in your refrigerator to things as complex as puffballs or mushrooms.

Fungal spores are tiny bits of protoplasm surrounded by a thick wall. This makes them very resistant to heat, cold, or dryness, which explains why fungi can reproduce almost anywhere in the world, under almost any conditions. Fungi have also evolved extremely powerful enzymes that allow them to digest and live off of a great variety of different substances.

Most people believe that fungi are simply disease-causing or spoilage organisms that are found in unsanitary conditions. In truth, fungi can be very beneficial. Most of our antibiotics are derived from them, including penicillin. Without fungi, we would not have those marvelous Roquefort and Camembert cheeses or the wonderful mushrooms, morels, and truffles that many consider to be such delicacies. Since yeast are single-cell fungi, some of our most popular foods and beverages such as leavened bread, beer, wine, and other alcoholic beverages owe their presence to these organisms.

One of the first references to fungi or mold stressing their negative characteristics was made in the Bible, in Leviticus, chapter 13. This section of the Bible describes the instructions that the Lord gave to Moses to ensure that the Jews kept themselves clean, healthy, and holy. Verses 1–46 refer to the need to quarantine people with rashes and skin diseases. While all skin diseases are referred to as leprosy, the descriptions are more along the lines of a mildewy mold infection. From the great number of verses devoted to this subject, such as the details of diagnosis, quarantine procedures, and treatment, it appears clear that it was considered to be of great importance.

The remainder of the chapter (verses 47–59) describes the cleaning treatment that had to be carried out for clothing that was found to be contaminated with mildew. If the mildew could not be removed from the clothing after the treatment, it had to be burned.

13:49. . . . if the mark is greenish or reddish in the garment or in the leather, or in the warp or in the woof, or in any article of leather, it is a leprous mark and shall be shown to the priest.

13:50. Then the priest shall look at the mark and shall quarantine the article with the mark for seven days.

13:51. He shall then look at the mark on the seventh day; if the mark has spread in the garment, whether in the warp or in the woof, or in the leather, whatever the purpose for which the leather is used, the mark is a leprous malignancy, it is unclean.

13:52. So he shall burn the garment, whether the warp or the woof, in wool or in linen, or any article of leather in which the mark occurs, for it is a leprous malignancy; it shall be burned in the fire.

To put things into perspective, the Bible is not referring to a few T-shirts purchased for three dollars at the local Wal-Mart store. The production of wool and linen garments was a very time-consuming and expensive process at that time—so burning the clothing was a pretty dramatic gesture. The details are fascinating. The first step was to determine if the mildew had been controlled or if it was spreading. Only if the mildew was found to be contained could the garment be washed and sent for reexamination. In fact, some of the regulations would be quite normal today in any reputable laundry service.

13:53. But if the priest shall look, and indeed the mark has not spread in the garment, either in the warp or in the woof, or in any article of leather,

13:54. . . . then the priest shall order them to wash the thing in which the mark occurs and he shall quarantine it for seven more days.

13:55. After the article with the mark has been washed, the priest shall again look, and if the mark has not changed its appearance, even though the mark has not spread, it is unclean; you shall burn it in the fire, whether an eating away has produced bareness on the top or on the front of it.

13:56. Then if the priest looks, and if the mark has faded after it has been washed, then he shall tear it out of the garment or out of the leather, whether from the warp or from the woof.

13:57. . . . and if it appears again in the garment, whether in the warp or in the woof, or in any article of leather, it is an outbreak; the article with the mark shall be burned in the fire.

Leviticus, chapter 14, goes on to describe the curative treatment for those people found to have "leprosy." Some of the cure seems a bit strange (killing a bird and dipping a live bird in the dead bird's blood, etc.). However, another aspect fits modern hygiene practices very well: wash clothes, shave hair, delay a week before entering the home. Just before entering the home, the individual must again shave off all hair, including beard, eyebrows, and so on—everything—and then wash once again.

In chapter 14, verses 33–48, the Lord tells Moses that some of the dwellings in the land of Canaan may still contain a plague of leprosy that he had previously placed upon the land. Again, highly detailed descriptions of how to remove the green and red mold are described. All mold residues had to be carted off beyond the city limits. If the mold was persistent, then the entire dwellings—stone, timbers, mortar, and so on—all had to be destroyed and disposed of outside the city!

The extreme detail of these chapters shows the significance given to fungal contamination from earliest written history.

The significance of mold contamination did not lessen with time. In 431 BCE, a series of wars broke out between Athens and its adversary, Sparta. The Spartans were aided by their allies, the Peloponnesians, who regularly invaded the Attica territory of Athens and wreaked havoc on the surrounding agriculture and economy. Thucydides, who lived through the Peloponnesian Wars, described a deadly plague that reached Athens in 430 BCE. Since he suffered from the plague himself, his description of the symptoms is generally considered to be accurate. His work, *The Peloponnesian War 2*, states:

49.2. In other cases, however, there were no early clinical symptoms; but suddenly, first of all, an intense heat of the head and both redness and burning of the eyes seized perfectly healthy people.

The insides of the mouth, both throat and tongue, were bloody and emitted an abnormal and foul-smelling breath.

49.3. Next there was a development from the symptoms to sneezing and hoarseness. Before long the trouble descended to the chest accompanied by coughing. Whenever it settled in the stomach, it upset it, and there ensued the vomiting of every kind of bile named by physicians, along with a great deal of pain and discomfort.

49.4. In most cases there were bouts of dry retching which produced severe spasms. In some cases this was soon after the abatement of the previous symptoms, but in other cases it was much later still.

49.5. On the outside, the body was not unduly hot to the touch nor pale, but reddish and purple, and there were tiny blisters and open sores scattered upon it. But their insides burnt so much that patients could not endure contact with anything, even the lightest clothing or linen sheets, and preferred to be naked. Most of all they wanted to throw themselves into cold water constrained by a thirst which could not be quenched. It made no difference whether they drank much or little.

49.6. An inability to rest quietly and to sleep affected them without respite. During the period when the disease was at its height, the body was not wasted, but, surprisingly, resisted the distress. So people died with some strength left (most on the ninth or seventh day, from the internal heat). If they survived this, most died later from weakness because the disease descended to the bowels where there was severe ulceration along with uniformly fluid diarrhea.

This description of symptoms sounds very similar to that of a contemporary disease resulting from the consumption of contaminated grain. As noted, it is called Alimentary Toxic Aleukia, or ATA. With these words, Thucydides described the terrible effects that an organism as basic as the lowly fungus could have on the course of human history.

Food has always played an important role in the great medical writings of the ancient Greek and Roman world. In addition to espousing the health benefits that foods provide, such writings also describe the poisonous or noxious effects of certain plants found throughout nature. What was totally unknown was the effects of invisible contaminating microorganisms on foods and the morbid diseases that they caused.

While a number of books in the Bible describe the significance of eating clean, uncontaminated foods, the justification given had much more to do with the maintenance of holiness rather than the preservation of health. Galen, a Greek physician, was the first highly regarded medical authority to formulate the notion that spoiled food, grain in particular, could be the origin of major diseases.

> In my opinion, bad foods are those which are so by nature, as, for example, . . . (there) . . . which we call wild plants; as well as barley and wheat and all the other cereals, which are good by nature, but which, due to putridity, have come to resemble those considered to be defective by nature, insofar as they have a tendency to become putrid after a long period of time, or have become filled with putridity because they have been wrongly stored, or have been attacked by fungi (erysibe) in the course of their growth. Thus, of the many people who are forced to eat such food in times of famine, some died from a putrid or pestilential fever, others as seized by a scabby (itching) and leprosy-like skin condition.[1]

EVENT 8. ST. ANTHONY'S FIRE

Most people have never heard of ergotism, much less the mold that causes it, *Claviceps purpurea*. This fungus starts life out as a small, black rind-covered tube called a sclerotium. Barely more than half an inch long and an eighth of an inch wide, this harmless-looking tube is

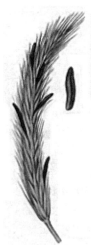

Claviceps purpurea, taken from Dennis E. Jackson, *Experimental Pharmacology and Materia Medica* (St. Louis: C. V. Mosby, 1939).

easily mistaken for a broken piece of plant stalk and would likely go totally unnoticed lying on the winter ground. Within its thick walls, however, a compact mass of mycelium lies dormant, awaiting the proper time to awake.

With the arrival of spring, the sclerotium awakens and sprouts a dozen or more stalks that looked like tiny enoki mushrooms. The heads of these stalks produce and discharge spores that are light enough to be carried by the passing winds. If they land on cereals, they quickly colonize them and produce a new sclerotium at every infection site.

Because the sclerotia resemble the spur of a rooster's leg, they were called "ergot" by the French.

The cereals most commonly affected are wheat, barley, rye, and oats—all common staples of the Western diet. As can be seen from the illustration, it would be quite easy to harvest the sclerotium along with the rest of the grain. According to agricultural records, in cold, damp periods, as much as a quarter of the harvest could be made up of ergot sclerotia! (Fortunately, this is no longer a significant problem because of improved postharvest practices and access to hot-air drying.)

Manually culling out these contaminants is a very time-consuming job, and it is not surprising that a considerable amount of ergot eventually becomes mixed in with the rest of the cereal grains. What makes matters worse is that the *Claviceps* continues to thrive if the moisture content exceeds 14 percent—a situation not uncommon in grain storage. Once the grain is removed from storage and milled into flour, it is very difficult to tell that a product is toxic. Aside from some slight discoloration, ergot-contaminated flour looks exactly like normal flour.

Ergot toxins are alkaloids (nitrogenous plant chemicals) that have profound effects on the central nervous system. Many of them are very powerful hallucinogens, including lysergic acid diethylamide, more commonly known as LSD. Aside from causing hallucinations, these toxins can severely contract arteries (vasoconstrictor) and smooth muscles, causing numbness, extreme sensitivity, and irritability.

In ancient times, the Chinese, Greeks, and Romans actually used ergot for its medicinal properties. A tea-like infusion from infected rye was used to reduce or stop postpartum hemorrhaging or to stop the bleeding of severe wounds. The vasoconstrictor function of the alkaloid ergotamine was even used to induce abortions. As a result, whenever flour contaminated with ergot was consumed unknowingly, the odds of miscarriage were increased enormously.

Ergotism manifests itself in two distinct ways. The first is called gangrenous ergotism, and the second is known as convulsive ergotism. Sometimes, both conditions can be found in the same victim.

Historically, gangrenous ergotism is more prominent, having been responsible for the infamous affliction St. Anthony's Fire. In this terrible manifestation of ergot-induced vasoconstriction, the limbs and their extremities (fingers and toes) become swollen and highly inflamed. Victims experience sensations of extreme heat (the "Holy Fire"). Within a few weeks, gangrene sets in and the fingers, toes, or limbs become necrotic and fall off. As can be imagined, this whole process was agonizingly painful because the limbs felt like they were consumed by fire.

Ergotism has been a regular curse to rye- and other grain-eating populations for millennia. It was first described in an Assyrian tablet as a "noxious pustule in the ear of grain." The ancient Egyptians were aware of a disease caused by eating certain grains that produced both convulsions and hallucinations. In 875 CE, the "Annals of Xanthes" described how "a great plague of swollen blisters consumed the people by a loathsome rot so that their limbs were loosened and fell off before death."[2] It was the first report of a mass outbreak of ergotism.

Another European ergot epidemic appeared in the eleventh century and was christened *ignis sacer* (Latin for "holy fire").[3] Although less common in England than in the rest of Europe, a number of major outbreaks of ergotism were recorded there in 1762 and 1734. In Russia, ergotism was a major health hazard, particularly in times of famine when little choice was left but to consume even blighted grain.

Out of desperation, victims prayed to their various saints for relief. One of the most popular saints was St. Anthony. Born in Alexandria, Egypt, in 251 CE, Anthony came from a wealthy family. At a young age, he gave all his wealth to the poor and banished himself to the desert where he became a hermit. He eventually migrated to Europe where he lived to the ripe old age of 105.

After his death, Anthony was secretly buried on his mountain retreat. However, in the year 561, his remains were discovered and moved back to Alexandria. After the city was sacked by Saracens in 1070, his remains were transferred to Constantinople (Istanbul). When the city was captured by the Crusaders, the emperor of Constantinople presented a member of the French nobility the remains of St. Anthony, which were promptly transported to the church of La Motte near Vienne, France.

In 1089 there was a terrible plague of ergotism in the French town of La Motte. A nobleman and his son were among those stricken, but in time, both were miraculously cured by what they believed were the magical powers of the ancient relics of St. Anthony housed in their local church. The nobleman, Gaston, and his son, Girond, soon pledged themselves and their estate to establish a hospital near the church. Since that time, gangrenous ergotism, previously called the Holy Fire, became commonly known as St. Anthony's Fire.

More than one hundred major outbreaks of St. Anthony's Fire have been reported with as many as forty thousand deaths attributed to a single incident that occurred in the year 944 in France. Despite our knowledge of the disease and the toxins that cause it, we continue to experience outbreaks. In the twentieth century, at least four major outbreaks occurred in the Soviet Union (1926), Ireland (1929), France (1951), and Ethiopia (1978).

The 1951 outbreak occurred in the small French village of Pont St. Esprit. This tiny town took its name from the old bridge that spanned the Rhône River. That year, France experienced one of its wettest summers in a very long time. The conditions were ideal for the development of *Claviceps*, and in mid-August, one of the town's two bakers noticed that the new batch of flour he used to make his baguettes was slightly grayer than the flour he normally used. Since flour distribution was a government monopoly at the time, he felt he had no choice but to use the flour he was given.

Within a day, more than two hundred of the villagers, all of whom purchased his baguettes, became very ill with what appeared to be food poisoning. Several people began to complain of lightheadedness, nausea, vomiting, vertigo, and diarrhea. In spite of the village's typical summer heat, people felt like they were freezing. Soon, people started going berserk, screaming through the night that they were being attacked by terrible apparitions. The hallucinations made people jump out of windows, claiming that they were on fire or that they could fly like airplanes.

The likely cause of this was the baguettes made with ergot-contaminated flour. Symptoms of both the gangrenous and the convulsive forms of ergotism combined to produce an epidemic that was so bizarre and frightening that the outbreak captured the French newspaper headlines for weeks. It took some time before the consulting physicians brought in to analyze the problem noticed a resemblance between the ongoing difficulties in the town and epidemics of ergot poisoning that had occurred more than a century before. Others, including the police, thought that they were witnessing some form of mercury contamination—akin to Mad Hatter's disease. But the laboratory data eventually pointed to ergotism.

Before this incident ebbed, hundreds of villagers suffered weeks of unbearable sleeplessness and hallucinations. Four of them died agonizing deaths. It was months before the village of Pont St. Esprit returned to a semblance of normal life. The memory of *le pain maudit* (the accursed bread) still remains.

NOTES

1. Galen, *De differentiis febrium*, book 1, chapter 4, from E. Lieber, "Galen on Contaminated Cereals as a Cause of Epidemics," *Bulletin of the History of Medicine* 44 (1970): 332–45.

2. "Some Facts about History," http://www.dimok.de/ergot/history.html (accessed August 28, 2006).

3. "Ignis Sacer, Holy Fire," http://www.botgard.ucla.edu/html/botany textbooks/economicbotany/Claviceps/ (accessed August 28, 2006).

PART III
EARLY MODERN TIMES

CHAPTER 4
THE RENAISSANCE AND THE ENLIGHTENMENT
(1300–1750 CE)

I f you were to look up the foods that were commonly consumed in the medieval and Renaissance periods, it is likely that you would come across a marvelous variety of animals roasted on the spit of the castle's kitchen, several types of fish taken from the pristine streams that flowed through the great estates, fragrant sauces made from herbs cultivated in the castle garden, and wine produced from the local vineyards. It all sounds idyllic, and these foods may have been the fare for a select few in the upper classes, but what really kept most people alive during this period were grains and legumes.

Grains supplied the basic carbohydrate calories, and peas and beans provided the complementary proteins required to sustain life. Two major technological developments allowed these two commodities to be produced in quantities sufficient to support the growth and development of a prosperous Europe. The first was the moldboard plow. This invention replaced the scratch plow, which was nothing more than a heavy stick scraped diagonally over the ground. This plow could do little more than scratch a shallow furrow in the soil (as its name implies). The moldboard plow was a significant improvement. It had three working parts: a strong metal blade that dug vertically into the carth; another blade that cut the earth horizontally at the grass-roots level; and behind both of these, a curve-shaped board that lifted and turned the cut slices of soil neatly over to one side.

The moldboard plow was ideally suited for the heavy soils of northern Europe; thus, large areas of formerly unused land could now be cultivated. The increase in food production resulted in a corresponding increase in population and wealth. In addition to the new plow, a new system of field crop rotation was developed that significantly boosted agricultural production. Three-field rotation—that is, one field planted at the end of the season with wheat or rye; the second field planted in spring with peas and lentils, beans, or barley; and the third field left fallow—allowed the land to be productive for two years out of three rather than one out of two, as had been the practice in the past. This created an immediate increase of 50 percent output.

The sketch of the heavy plow below is taken from a thirteenth-century Lincolnshire manuscript. In typical medieval fashion, the drawing has no perspective; however, it is not difficult to picture what the plow would have been like. The handles, the draw pole, and the yoke are actually parallel to the ground, while the rest of the plow is perpendicular to the ground.

The plow shown here would have been used with two draft ani-

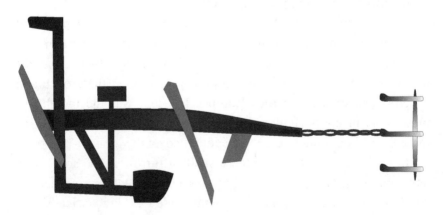

Thirteenth-century heavy plow,
image prepared by Morton Satin.

European Population (in millions) 650–1450 CE			
Place/Period	650	1000	1340	1450
Greece/Balkans	3	5	6	4.5
Italy	2.5	5	10	7.3
Spain/Portugal	3.5	7	9	7
Total—South	9	17	25	19
France/Low countries	3	6	19	12
British Isles	0.5	2	5	3
Germany/Scandinavia	2	4	11.5	7.3
Total—West/Central	5.5	15	35.5	22.5
Russia	2	6	8	6
Poland	1	2	3	2
Hungary	0.5	1.5	2	1.5
Total—East	3.5	9.5	13	9.3
TOTAL EUROPE	18	38.5	73.5	50

mals, such as horses or oxen. The yoke is attached to the plow by the draw chain.[1] The plow turned over the ground more vigorously, and with improvements in animal collars allowed hitherto noncultivatable land to be put into production. The increase in output of grain resulted in a population explosion.

The following table is a compilation of population estimates that reflected the ability of Europe to sustain the population increase.[2]

Although the population movement in each country varies some-what from the others, the general pattern is similar throughout all of Europe. In the three hundred and fifty years from 650 CE to 1000 CE the European population doubled as a result of the revolution in agriculture. A good deal of this can be attributed to the increase in agricultural output brought on by what is called the Medieval Warm Period—a phase of exceptionally warm weather in Europe that lasted from the tenth to the fourteenth century. The population doubled once more from 1000 to 1340 CE. Again, this second spurt in population growth was due to the tremendous increase in Western European grain output as a result of the weather and the adoption of improved agricultural technologies.

Unfortunately, this population explosion was cut short in the early fourteenth century as a result of several disastrous events. Political instability led to a European-wide recession toward the end of the thirteenth century. This was quickly followed by the onset of very bad weather in the opening years of the fourteenth century. Cold, damp weather dramatically reduced the yields of grain throughout Europe and initiated a series of calamitous famines throughout the breadth of the continent with sporadic local famines occurring on a regular basis.

In the years 1315–1317, what became know as the Great Famine ravaged all of Europe. It started with a wet spring in the year 1315. The rain-saturated soil made it all but impossible to plow the fields that were ready for cultivation. To make matters worse, the heavy rains rotted a large portion of the seeding grains before they could germinate properly. Throughout the spring and summer, the rains continued and the temperature remained cool. Not surprisingly, the annual harvest was much smaller than usual, resulting in a rapid depletion of the very meager food reserves kept by most families.

In order to survive, peasants went out into the forests to gather whatever food they could find: roots, mushrooms, ground plants, grass, nuts, and even bark to supplement their meager and moldy grain supplies. Ravaged by malnutrition, the rural populations, who did almost all the work, were severely weakened. The following spring and summer of 1316 were once again cold and wet. Peasant workers, depleted of the sheer physical energy needed to till the heavy, wet soil, used up their food supplies to a point where they could no longer sustain them until the next harvest.

It has been estimated that more than 10 percent of the population perished during these famines. This period was soon followed by the bubonic plague, or Black Death, which broke out in 1347. In the ninety years from 1350 to 1440, the population of Europe did not increase; on the contrary, it decreased by 30 percent.

EVENT 9. IN WITCH MOLD WAS SALEM CAST?

From the earliest written histories, the combination of symptoms experienced by ergotism victims led them to believe that they were cursed by supernatural powers. Such sentiments easily led to the assumption that witches must be involved in the disease. In fact, nurses and midwives, who routinely lived under the suspicion of being witches because of their keen knowledge of nature, had to be particularly careful during epidemic outbreaks.

The most famous witch-related incidents in the United States were the Salem witch trials that took place in the year 1692. The reason for these trials has been debated for over three centuries. There is no doubt that local politics, puritanical values, religious paranoia, greed, jealousy, and a healthy dose of adolescent imagination all played a role in bringing about these trials, but perhaps there were other factors moldering about.

Salem was a town divided. In the western part of the village were the farmers—strong, hardy folk who were heavily steeped in Puritan traditions. The residents of the eastern side of the village were associated with the rich harbor economy and, as a result, were far more modern in their outlook on life and the toleration of other cultures.

It was in this charged climate in December 1691 that eight girls, including the daughter and niece of the minister of the western part of town, Rev. Samuel Parris, became afflicted with convulsive fits and bizarre behavior. The local physicians could not explain away these symptoms, although in February 1692, one suggested the possibility that the girls were bewitched. He planted this malicious seed in fertile soil; the Puritans were great believers in witches and the harm that they could bring to a community. After this doctor's pronouncement, events began to unfold rapidly.

One of the village women, Mary Sibley, asked the Reverend Parris's Barbados slave, Tituba, and her husband to bake a "witch cake," made from rye meal and urine from the victims, in order to help the girls reveal their tormentors. In due course, the girls named Tituba and two older village women as the culprits. On February 29, Leap Day, the three women were taken into custody immediately after charges had been made against them.

The strange behavior of the girls continued, and a full-blown witch hunt ensued, snaring both men and women. An outbreak of smallpox, the constant fear of Indian attacks, and the unending difficulties of survival in a harsh, new land fed the anxiety that drove the accusations. Misfortune was often attributed to the works of the devil, and at this moment in Salem's history, witches had to be found.

By the end of May 1692, over two hundred people had been jailed on suspicion of being involved in witchcraft. The new royal governor, William Phips, recently dispatched from England, established a special court that, by June 2, began hearing cases.

Justice worked quickly in Puritan America. The first trial and consequent conviction led to the hanging of Bridget Bishop on June 10. In the next three months, an additional eighteen men and women were hanged and one man was crushed to death by stone weights. The key evidence was the girls' descriptions of apparitions of the accused. Of all the people accused, only those who maintained their innocence were executed. Those who confessed their sins were considered worthy of being spared. It is no great surprise that all the accusers came from the west, or the poorer end of the village, while almost all of the accused came from the east side. Envy and hatred had found an ideal outlet.

When trying to interpret the events in a modern light, it is tempting to say that the accusing girls simply drove themselves into a state of hysteria. The problem with this explanation is that the well-documented records appear to describe symptoms severe enough to be virtually impossible to fake.

A connection between the strange behavior of the Salem girls and convulsive ergotism was first made by Linnda Caporael in 1960.[3] Putting together evidence regarding the crops consumed, the growing conditions, the timing of the critical events, and the symptoms of the victims, Caporael developed a very credible case implicating ergotism as the causative factor that led to the Salem witch trials.

This theory has been challenged as well as supported by more thorough analysis.[4] Like so many other episodes from our past, there is simply not enough evidence to readily confirm or deny this theory with certainty. The potential for ergotism to have been a mitigating factor certainly did exist. All of Salem's accusers did not necessarily have to ingest high levels of ergot. There are several cases of mass hysteria brought on by one or two people with verifiable symptoms, while the remaining group may have simply got caught up in the ensuing excitement.

By mid-September, the witch-hunting frenzy waned, and although several other indictments were handed down into the court, no one else was executed. By May 1693, the royal governor granted a general reprieve, and all one hundred and fifty witches remaining in custody were released, thus ending an extraordinary, albeit shameful, chapter in the nation's young life.

Another fungal contaminant of grain is the *Fusarium* mold, a filamentous fungi that is widely distributed in soil and closely associated with plants. Like *Claviceps*, *Fusarium* has an established and prominent place in the history of European morbidity and mortality. *Fusarium* species are responsible for blights, root rots, and cankers in legumes, grains, and grasses.

The role of *Fusaria* as a potent producer of mycotoxins remained unsuspected until the 1970s. Since that time, however, research has firmly established its role in major episodes of human mycotoxicosis (poisoning by mold toxins). Its prominent position in the fungal rogue's gallery is a result of the three different kinds of toxins it produces.

The first toxin, zearalenone, is a chemical that causes severe deformations to reproductive organs by imitating the estrogen hormone.

The second toxin, fumosin, can cause severe and irreversible damage to organs and has been implicated in esophageal cancer. The third and most deadly toxins produced by the *Fusarium* mold are called trichlothecenes, one of which, dubbed T-2, is the most notorious of all.

If consumed by humans, the T-2 toxin can result in a condition first described by the Russians in 1943 as Alimentary Toxic Aleukia, or ATA. When infected by *Fusarium*, a wide range of grains including rice, rye, wheat, barley, corn, and millet can produce T-2 toxins capable of causing ATA. An epidemic in the USSR killed an estimated one hundred thousand people between 1942 and 1948.[5] It is now known that ATA also occurred in Russia in 1932 and before that in 1913, and there is little doubt that outbreaks occurred in earlier years as well.

The pathological course of ATA development in humans is both strange and terrible. When infected grain is consumed, victims first experience headache, vomiting, throat inflammation, and gastroenteritis. Then, the symptoms subside even if contaminated grain continues to be part of the diet.

But the T-2 toxin acts like a time bomb. Victims can continue consuming infected grains without noticing overt symptoms for anywhere from two weeks to two months. And during that time, the T-2 toxins continue to exert their effects. The T-2 toxin kills bone marrow stem cells, causing the destruction and shrinkage of bone marrow. The end result is a massive immune deficiency characterized by considerable ulceration of the digestive tract, as well as pulmonary hemorrhages. Once diagnosed, the body has suffered too much damage to be able to fight back. Mortality rates from ATA are very high.

During World War II, tens of thousands of Russians—most, but not exclusively, located in the Orenburg district close to the Caspian Sea—perished from ATA because they were forced to consume grain infected with *Fusarium* mold. More recently, in the Zhejiang province of China, a small epidemic broke out after people ate rice contaminated with *Fusarium* toxins. As in all the outbreaks, rainy weather and poor storage conditions led to the *Fusarium* contamination.[6]

Professor Mary Kilborne Matossian has constructed a well-documented and plausible theory that mold poisoning played a critical role in repressing population growth in England (and perhaps elsewhere in Europe) between the sixteenth and nineteenth centuries.[7] Basing her research on factors such as population figures, child mortality, and fever epidemic, she convincingly argues that ergotism and ATA were critical factors in child mortality and the consequent reduction in European population growth with all its consequent social impacts.

It is interesting to note that, unlike England, Ireland did not experience the same child mortality rates during the same period because that country's staple food was potatoes rather than grain. Unfortunately, another fungus, *Phytophthora infestans*, devastated the Irish potato crop in 1845. This blight caused the country's population to plummet from eight million to less than five million because of starvation, disease, and emigration. The Irish Famine of 1846–1950 totally changed the social and political structure of Ireland, and Irish emigration had a lasting impact on the political life of the United States that continues through today, a century and a half later.

Silent, unobtrusive, and seldom the focus of our thoughts, the lowly fungus among us has had a far greater impact on our history and social evolution than most of our most famous historical figures and events.

EVENT 10. WHAT BUGGED LITTLE LOUIS

In 1671 Prince Louis II invited King Louis XIV (aka Louis the Great, the Sun King, Little Louis) to his beautiful chateau at Chantilly. He told his illustrious chef, Vatel, to prepare a reception for the king and his entourage of two hundred guests. Vatel thought this was a grand opportunity to impress the king with his extraordinary cuisine.

On Friday morning, April 24, while everyone was still asleep, Vatel anxiously awaited a large shipment of fish he had ordered for the feast. When only two small loads arrived, he became very distraught. "My honor is lost; this is a humiliation that I cannot endure." He could not help but to envision Louis the Great and his many courtesans sitting down to plates that were void of food. He scribbled down a brief note: "The shame is too much to bear." Vatel then retired to his room, jammed his sword against the door, and ran it through his heart three times. He fell dead at the very same time that the rest of the fish for the feast arrived, as ordered. In honor of Vatel's memory, the filet of sole that he planned to serve was dropped from the menu.[8]

Such were the heights to which culinary genius was cherished during the reign of the Sun King.

This view of cuisine as an art form was continued and elaborated on by Jean Anthelme Brillat-Savarin, the celebrated eighteenth-century French politician and gastronome. He felt that the discovery of a new dish conferred more happiness to humanity than the discovery of a new star. In his book *Physiologie du Goût*, Brillat-Savarin wrote, "Tell me what you eat and I will tell you what you are." This has been usually truncated to "You are what you eat" and refers to the way in which foods and their nutrients affect your health and well-being.

Brillat-Savarin could also have said, "Tell me what's eating you and I will tell you who you are," but the origin of foodborne parasites was unknown during his lifetime. If he had said such a thing, recent research indicates that he would have been quite correct, because in the sixteenth to eighteenth centuries, where you were on the socio-economic scale had a great bearing on the parasites you harbored. Surprisingly, the higher up the social ladder you were, the more foodborne parasites you were bound to be infected with.

Proof of this extraordinary little detail comes from a small but highly specialized group of experts who study ancient latrine sediments and coprolites collected from archaeological sites preserved by natural conditions. From these remains, it is possible to ascertain some of the diseases suffered by those that produced them. This research is based on the identification of parasite eggs through their microscopic morphology, in addition to a knowledge of the biological cycles of the modern incarnations of these parasites. The results reveal the kinds of foods consumed as well as the sanitation conditions that were prevalent at the time.

Louis XIV ruled France for seventy-two years (1643–1715)—longer than any other major European monarch. In order to get away from the swarm of courtiers and advisers at Versailles, Little Louis decided he needed a small retreat with some solitude. He eventually found a narrow valley not far from Versailles that was almost unapproachable because of marshes and hills surrounding it on all sides. On one slope was a small, wretched village called Marly. That is where he decided to build.

Not unexpectedly, his small refuge, called Marly-le-Roi, soon began to expand. Building after building sprang up, the surrounding hills were flattened, and formal gardens with fantastic waterworks were constructed. In his *Memoirs* of life at Court, the Duc de Saint-Simon, a contemporary of Louis XIV, stated that Marly-le-Roi ended up costing more than Versailles! No wonder the seeds of the French Revolution were planted as soon as Louis XIV died.

Marly-le-Roi and the despotic rule it represented were wiped out during the Revolution. On a cold day in October 1789, the Revolutionary mobs dragged Louis XVI out of his palace in Versailles to the Tuileries Palace in Paris. A few years later (1793), he was obliged to visit the guillotine on Place de la Concorde in Paris. The fever of the Revolution destroyed Marly-le-Roi so completely that nothing remains except a few small roads, several trees, and the original horse pond.

Recent archaeological excavations uncovered the site of Marly-le-Roi's latrines, which were constructed in 1680 and used continuously until Louis XIV's death in 1715. The unique construction of the latrines did not allow contamination from other sources and so any parasite remains found in the sediments would be specifically associated with the king and his courtiers. This unique discovery called for paleoarchaeologists par excellence.

Dr. Françoise Boucher, professor of parasitology in the faculty of medicine at Reims, together with a team of experts from France's National Center for Scientific Research, was called to investigate the remnants in Marly-le-Roi's latrines.[9] The team's meticulous analyses provided an excellent insight into the parasitic diseases that the Sun King and his courtiers suffered from.

The two most prevalent types of parasite eggs were the round-worms *Ascaris* and *Trichuris*, species that are still a problem today. *Ascaris* is a large roundworm found in humans, pigs, and some other animals. (*Ascaris lumbricoides* is the parasite found in humans, while *Ascaris suum* infects pigs and wild boars.) While these worms normally range from six to twelve inches in length and are usually about a quarter inch in diameter, specimens as large as sixteen inches long have been recovered. *Ascaris* is spread through the ingestion of their tiny eggs. A female *Ascaris* worm may contain as many as twenty-five thousand microscopic eggs at any time and can eliminate as many as two hundred thousand per day into the host's intestine. The eggs are then spread in human and animal waste.

Symptoms of *Ascaris* infection are abdominal pains, vomiting, nausea, and a protruding abdomen. Once ingested, the larvae burrow into tissues, where they can cause severe damage. As they grow, they seek out the body's intestinal tract and lodge there to produce more eggs. On occasion, they can even crawl up the throat and out the mouth or nose. We'll learn more about this in event 20, "Bioterrorism and the Food Supply" in chapter 6.

Trichuris trichiura, a roundworm that is fairly common in Europe, is notable for its small size compared to *Ascaris lumbricoides*. The worm derives its name from its characteristic whiplike shape, with adults reaching a length of one and a half to two inches. The *Trichuris* buries its thin front end into the intestinal mucosa and feeds on tissue secretions, not blood. This worm does not migrate through the tissues like the *Ascaris* and therefore does not cause as much damage, although heavy infections can result in similar symptoms.

Trichuris is found in other animals, which can serve as alternate sources of infection. The use of unsterilized "night soil," which contains both types of parasite eggs, as a fertilizer, is a definite cause of reinfection and the reason why this parasite is found on fresh vegetables. Humans are infected by this type of produce if it is consumed raw.

In addition to *Ascaris* and *Trichuris*, Boucher and his colleagues found encapsulated tapeworm embryos, but were unable to differentiate between beef- and pork-derived varieties (*Taenia saginata* and *Taenia solium*). Adult tapeworms have an average length of fifteen feet but may grow to fifty feet in length. They don't come trailing out of the normal twenty-five-foot human intestine (as one of my fellow students once asked) but are folded over in several sections. Adult tapeworms are flat and are characterized by the presence of a small head, which has rows of tiny hooks for attaching to the intestine of the host. Right behind the head is a narrow neck, followed by flat, rectangular-shaped body segments. These segments contain both testes and ovaries and continually produce eggs. The body segments farthest from the head and closest to the end of the intestine develop most rapidly. Once they are mature, the segments separate from the rest of the worm and pass out with the feces of their host. These segments contain numerous eggs, which are simply encapsulated embryonic tapeworms waiting for a new host to release them. Humans are usually infected by ingestion of undercooked or raw meat.

The symptoms of infection with beef tapeworms (*T. saginata*) are variable. Many infections are completely asymptomatic, but in other cases they can be serious as a result of intestinal blockage.

Pork tapeworm (*Taenia solium*) infections are another story. The embryos hatch in the intestine and bore their way into the tissues to form cysts known as cysticerci. This cysticercosis state is the most dangerous form of tapeworm disease because of the tissues the larvae invade and damage. The hatched tapeworm embryos can burrow their way to the eyes, lungs, liver, heart, and brain of the victim, wreaking inflammatory havoc and infection all along the way. The most serious form of this disease is cerebral (neurocysticercosis), which often leads to epilepsy and death. The annual worldwide cysticercosis mortality has been estimated at approximately fifty thousand cases.

Boucher and his group found another parasite that infested the king's court, *Fasciola hepatica*, the liver fluke, which was most likely ingested by consuming fresh watercress and dandelion greens. Adult parasites have a flat leaflike body about an inch long and a half inch wide.

After ingestion, the cysts hatch in the small intestine and release the young parasite. They then penetrate the gut wall, entering the peritoneal cavity. The *Fasciola hepatica* then migrates directly to the liver, where it penetrates and damages the tissue. The infection is rarely fatal and causes fairly nonspecific symptoms including an intermittent fever, mild jaundice, and in some cases anemia.

Fresh vegetables—available to the wealthy—were rarely consumed by the poor. The presence of *Ascaris*, *Trichuris*, and *Fasciola* are strong indicators of poor hygiene during the preparation of vegetables and salads, not particularly surprising, since the knowledge of transmission of pathogenic organisms was very limited. The presence of *Taenia* cysts confirms the contamination of meat and its consumption in an uncooked or almost raw state. Poor people did not suffer from this parasite because they had so little meat that it was usually boiled in a soup with coarse grains and starchy vegetables.

As a result of the accessibility of both fresh vegetables and meat, royalty was far more prone to chronic parasitic infections than the poor. These parasitic diseases sapped the physical and mental strength of the victims and often left them in a chronic state of pain and agitation—a condition not conducive to making wise judgments. And it was the royalty and the upper classes who created the policies that resulted in the events that made history.

NOTES

1. Paul J. Gans, 1997–2002, http://scholar.chem.nyu.edu/tekpages/heavyplow.html (accessed June 5, 2006).

2. Paul Halsall, 1996, http://www.fordham.edu/halsall/source/pop-in-eur.html (accessed June 5, 2006).

3. L. R. Caporael, "Ergotism: The Satan Loosed in Salem?" *Science* 192 (April 2, 1976): 21–26.

4. N. P. Spanos and J. Gottlieb, "Ergotism and the Salem Witch Trials," *Science* 194 (December 24, 1976): 1390–94; N. P. Spanos, "Ergotism and the Salem Witch Panic," *Journal of the History of Behavioral Science* 19 (October 1983): 358–69; M. K. Matossian, "Ergot and the Salem Witchcraft

Affair," *American Scientist* 70 (July–August 1982): 355–57; M. K. Matossian, *Poisons of the Past* (New Haven, CT: Yale University Press, 1989).

5. A. Z. Joffe, "Fusarium Poae and F. Sporotrichioides as Principal Causal Agents of Alimentary Toxic Aleukia," in *Mycotoxic Fungi, Mycotoxins, Mycotoxicoses: An Encyclopaedic Handbook*, vol. 3, ed. T. D. Wyllie and L. G. Morehouse (New York: Marcel Dekker, 1978), pp. 21–86.

6. J. N. Feng and Z. G. Wang, "Food Poisoning Caused by Moldy Rice Contaminated with Fusarium and T-2 Toxin," *Chinese Journal of Preventative Medicine* 26, no. 5 (1992): 284–86.

7. M. K. Matossian, "Mold Poisoning: An Unrecognized English Health Problem, 1550–1800," *Medical History* 25 (1981): 73–84.

8. *Rogov's Ramblings*, "Liberte, Egalite, Gastronomie or No Need for Suicide," http://www.stratsplace.com/rogov/no_need_suicide.html (accessed August 28, 2006).

9. F. Bouchet, "Recovery of Helminth Eggs from Archaeological Excavations of the Grand Louvre (Paris, France)," *Journal of Parasitology* 80 (1995): 785–86; F. Bouchet et al., "The First Recovery of *Schistosoma mansoni* Eggs from a Latrine in Europe (15th–16th Century)," *Journal of Parasitology* 88 (2002): 404–405; A. Cockburn et al., "Autopsy of an Egyptian Mummy," *Science* 187 (1975): 1155–60; B. Herrmann, "Parasite Remains from Mediaeval Latrine Deposits: An Epidemiologic and Ecologic Approach," *Note et monographie technique* n°24, CNRS, Paris (1988): 135–42.

PART IV
THE MODERN ERA

CHAPTER 5

THE INDUSTRIAL REVOLUTION

(1750–1900 CE)

The beginning of the Industrial Revolution was characterized by the development of mechanized agriculture, which drove many rural laborers off the farm and into the squalid workhouses of the cities. The increased demand for food to feed urban workers and for raw materials to keep the factories running resulted in a total realignment of production and trade patterns. In particular, the concentration of agricultural production, processing, and trade migrated into the hands of fewer and larger enterprises, which ended up establishing the conditions for the mass food poisonings that were to be regularly experienced over the next two centuries.

The increasing demand for foods that would not readily spoil prompted the development of new food-processing technologies such as canning that are still in use today. Initial efforts to preserve foods resulted in a great deal of food poisoning simply because no one understood the mechanism behind successful preservation. It was only in the last half of the nineteenth century that the scientific basis for food and beverage spoilage became understood—largely because of the work of Louis Pasteur. This knowledge quickly ushered in an era of understanding that led to new technologies that revolutionized food production and processing in the twentieth century.

EVENT 11. VOYAGE OF THE DAMNED— FROM CANS TO CANNIBALS!

Any review of Egyptian hieroglyphics, Bible verses, ancient Greek or Roman texts, or the current volumes of *Food Science and Technology* will readily confirm that the preservation of food has always been a major preoccupation.

Perhaps the most significant development in the history of food preservation was the process of canning. As with most other innovations, canning did not arise spontaneously. Other ideas and experiences with food preservation had been tried and documented. By the middle of the eighteenth century, it was generally accepted that the spoilage of certain foods could be slowed down through the use of heat. The problem was that no one had any idea why heat worked so well, because the concept of microbial spoilage still remained undiscovered.

Toward the end of the eighteenth century, Napoleonic France was the powerhouse of Europe. The Society for the Encouragement of National Industry (Société d'Encouragement pour l'Industrie Nationale) was extremely influential in fostering the types of research and development that could benefit the country's industry, agriculture, and trade.

The Société encouraged the public to submit their ideas and discoveries and made sure to reserve a prominent place for deserving entries in their famous "Bulletin." This not only ensured the rapid dissemination of new ideas and information but solicited an increasing input of more sophisticated experimental work.

Nicholas Appert (1749–1841), a Parisian confectioner, had developed a method to preserve certain foods in the 1790s. By the turn of the century, he had an operational factory at Massy (Seine et Oise) that apparently employed fifty people. It was the world's first canning plant—only it didn't use tin cans, it used glass bottles instead.

The key principles behind Appert's process were simple:

a. Put what you want to preserve into bottles.
b. Cork the bottles very carefully.

c. Place the corked bottles in a boiling water bath.

d. Remove the bottles from the water bath after the required period of time.

Simple, n'est-ce pas?

Using this technique, Appert produced the world's first canned foods and even sent them around the world with the French navy in 1806. His results were so impressive that the Société nominated a special committee just to review his process and products.

With one exception, the members of this blue ribbon committee approved Appert's work and products. Their only reservation was that they felt glass containers might not be practical because they were so easily broken. Appert, on the other hand, felt strongly that glass was the purest material he could use. He later said, "Je n'ai hasarde aucun essai d'autres matières" (I have not risked experiments with any other materials). The committee went on to encourage Appert to submit his new discovery to the Ministry of the Interior's Board of Arts and Manufactures.

Three years later, the ministry board rewarded him with a prize of twelve thousand francs and asked him to publish his work. In 1810, his now famous classic *Le Livre de tous les Ménages ou l'Art de Conserve pendant Plussiers Années Toutes les Substances Animales et Végétales* (The Art of Preserving All Kinds of Animals and Vegetable Substances for Several Years) was published.

Shortly after the publication of Appert's first book, a process obviously based on his invention was developed in England by John Hall and Bryan Donkin. It is possible that they paid Appert for the details of this process, because there is an indication in the company's historical records that John Hall and his associates paid £1,000 to "a French Patent biochemist named Appert."[1] This was somewhat odd, however, since Appert never patented his process and there is absolutely no record of this transaction in Appert's business accounts. It may very well be that Hall placed this note in his records as a form of protection in case he was asked where he got his process from.[2]

In any event, it is clear that the Hall-Donkin process was based on

THE ART

OF

PRESERVING

ALL KINDS OF

Animal and Vegetable Substances

FOR

SEVERAL YEARS.

———◆———

A WORK PUBLISHED BY ORDER OF THE

FRENCH MINISTER OF THE INTERIOR,

On the Report of the Board of Arts and Manufactures,

BY

M. APPERT.

———◆———

TRANSLATED FROM THE FRENCH.

═════

LONDON:

PRINTED FOR BLACK, PARRY, AND KINGSBURY,

BOOKSELLERS TO THE HON. EAST-INDIA COM-

PANY, LEADENHALL STREET.

———

1812.

Cover page of M. Appert, *The Art of Preserving All Kinds of Animal and Vegetable Substances for Several Years*, vol. 1 from the Mallinckrodt Collection of Food Classics. Facsimile of the 1812 edition (1966).

Appert's work. The processes differed in the material used as the food container; Hall and Donkin used iron canisters to replace Appert's glass bottles. Two other English patents by de Heine and Durand stressed the use of tin-plated iron canisters instead of glass. Because of the fragility of glass, cans were more practical and quickly became the favorite container for preserved foods. In fact, the 1818 French competition for food preservation by the Appert method sponsored by the Ministry of the Interior's Board of Arts and Manufactures only allowed for products in metal containers. The age of canning had begun in earnest.

Strangely enough, although commercial canning was firmly under way, the exact reason why canned foods did not spoil was still unknown. Of the different theories explaining why the process worked, the most widely held was that of the brilliant French chemist Joseph Louis Gay-Lussac. (He was famous for his law stating that the pressure of a fixed volume of gas will vary in proportion to the temperature.) In 1810, after analyzing Appert's products, Gay-Lussac concluded that the total absence of oxygen in the products was the reason why they didn't putrefy. Unfortunately, the true explanation was more than fifty years away. It was Pasteur who finally concluded that it was the heating process that destroyed the microorganisms responsible for food spoilage and disease.

It is interesting to note that the most pathogenic organism associated with canned products is *Clostridium botulinum*—the organism that causes botulism. Since it is an anaerobic microorganism, *Clostridium botulinum* can grow only in the absence of oxygen. If, as the renowned Gay-Lussac believed, the absence of oxygen was the key to canning, then canning would never have succeeded because a great many consumers would have succumbed to botulism. In fact, many attempts were made to eliminate or displace oxygen without heating: by bubbling nitrogen or hydrogen gas through the products or by placing them under a vacuum prior to sealing them. But these processes never worked. Fortunately, the successful experiences with heating the products for extended periods of time ensured that all the pathogenic and spoilage organisms were killed (even though the people that carried out the processing had no idea what was going on).

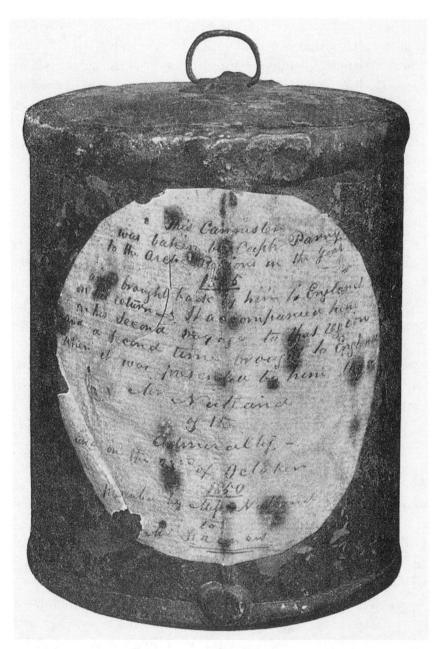

Old, hand-soldered can, taken from *Historic Tinned Foods Publication #85*, International Tin Research and Development Council (Middlesex, England: Greenfield, 1939).

"An army marches on its stomach"—attributed to Napoleon— highlights the importance of food for the proper functioning of the military. Notwithstanding the difficulties of keeping an army marching along, the navy had it much worse, because crew members were cut off from all sources of fresh food once they set sail. Scurvy and other nutrient-deficiency diseases killed and disabled far more soldiers and sailors than the epic sea battles ever did.

Prior to Appert's discovery, the most technologically advanced preserved food was a product called "portable soup." This abomination was made by first preparing a meat broth from the parts of the carcass that could not be put to better use. To limit rancidity, the fat was skimmed off to be used as tallow for making soap and candles. The remaining broth was boiled until almost all the liquid evaporated,

From "Meriwether Lewis Goes Shopping," *Calendar Features April 2004 Feature*, National Archives, http://www.archives.gov/ calendar/features/2004/04.htm/ (accessed July 28, 2005).

"having by long boiling evaporated the most putrescent parts of the meat, it is reduced to the consistence of glue, which in effect it is, and will like other glue in a dry place keep sound for years together."[3] In fact, portable soup was often adulterated with crude fish or beef glue to make it cheaper.[4] To make it easier to eat, the mixture was covered in blood and water until it dissolved into a soup. The gluelike nature of portable soup ensured that it was a product equally appreciated by both seamen and carpenters.

The famous explorer Captain Cook routinely fed his men one ounce of this concoction every week—an excellent excuse for mutiny if there ever was one. As can be seen in the accompanying note, Meriwether Lewis purchased 193 pounds of portable soup in 1803 for the legendary expedition across America, but the product proved to be so unpopular that it was consumed only when the explorers were close to starvation.[5]

Not surprisingly, canned and bottled foods proved to be in great demand after they became available in 1810. They were a great boon to the increasingly prolonged voyages that were made to explore the vast reaches of the globe. In 1818 the company of Donkin, Hall and Gamble supplied the British Admiralty with close to thirty thousand cans of various meat, vegetable, and soup products.

For those sailors heading south to the tropics, there was always the possibility of obtaining fresh food at the destination. However, if you were bound for the Arctic, that option was out of the question, hence the quantity and quality of shipboard food supplies were of paramount importance.

The first of the Arctic explorers to bring along canned goods was the Russian naval officer Otto von Kotzebue. Prior to his departure, he heard of "a discovery lately made in England," which he felt was "too important not to be made use of for the expedition."[6] On July 30, 1815, he set sail with twenty-seven men to find a passage through the Arctic Ocean. His experience with the "tin boxes" was far better than the traditional dried provisions he took upon the recommendation of the Economic Society of St. Petersburg—they all went bad!

The next Arctic expedition to carry canned foods was that of Sir

William Parry on his famous voyage to discover the Northwest Passage in 1819. Bryan Donkin's canned provisions formed a significant portion of the stores taken aboard the *Hecla* and the *Griper*, the two vessels Parry commanded. Parry found the food to be very suitable, in particular when they had to traverse Melville Island by sled. The surgeons of the two ships commented as follows:

H.M. Ship *Hecla*
December 9, 1820

... for my opinion of the preserved meats and soups supplied by Messers. Gamble and Co. . . . I beg leave to state that I consider them to have been acquisitions of the highest value. . . . I am also happy in testifying to the general good quality of those provisions as well as to the perfection of the antiseptic process employed by Messers. Gamble and Co. by which their meats and soups continue in an unimpaired state of preservation to the end of voyage. I have the honor to remain, etc.

(Sgd.) John Edwards,
Surgeon

———

H.M. Ship *Griper*
December 9, 1820

... The soups I consider peculiarly excellent, especially as I have every reason to believe that the antiscorbutic [antiscurvy] quality of the vegetable is not injured in its preparation. . . .

(Sgd.) C. I. Beverley,
Asst. Surgeon

It was clear that cans were an enormous improvement in the preservation of foods. The industry and the military were racing together full steam ahead as exemplified by the testimony of Captain Basil Hall, who described how appealing canned foods were to the navy in this entry from the *Encyclopedia Britannica*, 1841:

> It is really astonishing how good the preserved milk is . . . and you must, on examining the prices, bear in mind that meat thus preserved eats nothing, nor drinks—it is not apt to die—does not tumble overboard or get its legs broken . . . it takes no care in the keeping—it is always ready, may be eaten hot or cold, and this enables you to toss into a boat as many days' cooked provisions as you require. [Of course, he was referring to the common practice at the time of bringing live animals onboard as a source of fresh meat.]

In 1841 two very important canning developments were patented. The first was a British patent awarded to Hungarian-born Stephan Goldner wherein:

> a mode of heating the vessels in which animal or vegetable substances are to be preserved by driving off the atmospheric air and producing a vacuum therein, which has heretofore for the most part been performed by stoves or ovens which is liable to burn the materials. I employ a chemical bath in the manner described by John Wertheimer's Patent. I use a solution of muriate of lime or nitrate of soda, but prefer the former because I am enabled to obtain a constant temperature of 270–280°F without much evaporation.

The second patent, also British, was awarded to John Wertheimer, who, in addition to using a calcium chloride bath, employed a method of sealing the can aperture while the products were still in the process of being heated. In fact, it appears that both patents were based on a French patent previously awarded to Monsieur Andre Fastier in 1839, who used both a brine bath to raise the processing temperature and a "hot" sealing system. It seems obvious that the credit for the discovery of this great advance really belongs to the French rather than the British.

Each of the patents stressed the importance of removing the air from the cans. This understanding of why canning appeared to work was based on Gay-Lussac's original premise made in 1810. In 1840 no one had a clue that microorganisms could cause spoilage and disease, and Louis Pasteur was just starting his work at the time.

Stephan Goldner was an astute businessman who wanted to quickly exploit his patent commercially. He set up factories in Houndsditch near London and on the banks of the Danube in Galatz (Moldavia, Romania), offering a great variety of canned foods including milk, soups, turtle, carrots, and ox tongues. At the bottom of his long list of provisions is a statement indicating that he was able to supply canisters ranging in size from one pound to five hundred pounds each. (A five-hundred-pound canister would be equivalent to a sixty-gallon drum.)

The age of Queen Victoria's reign was one of remarkable achievement for the British Empire. England was at the zenith of her power and consistently demonstrated this in the arts, sciences, engineering, military, and commercial trade. John Barrow, the secretary of the navy, was concerned that Russian exploration in the Arctic by the likes of Otto von Kotzebue posed a military and commercial threat to the empire. Barrow wanted his navy to discover a northwest passage from the Atlantic to the Pacific—the shortest possible trade route to Asia. In 1818 Barrow sent an expedition to Baffin Island and Lancaster Sound but was unable to proceed any farther. The following year, Sir Edward Parry led another expedition that sailed farther west than anyone had previously and farther than anyone else would for the remainder of the century. Parry sailed as far as Melville Island, which lies along the same longitudinal meridian as the border between Saskatchewan and Alberta, Canada.

At the same time, the British Admiralty sent John Franklin overland from Hudson Bay to the mouth of the Coppermine River on the Arctic Ocean. There he was supposed to link up with Parry and then proceed together to Alaska (which was still Russian territory at the time). This did not work as planned, but Franklin did map a significant portion of Arctic coastline. Franklin ventured again to the Arctic in 1825 and carefully mapped another large chunk of territory. For his efforts, Franklin was knighted in 1829. He also received the honorary degree of DCL (Doctor of Civil Law) from the University of Oxford, the gold medal of the Geographical Society of Paris, and was elected corresponding member of the Paris Academy of Sciences.

In 1836 he accepted the governorship of Van Diemen's Land (Tasmania), a post he held until the end of 1843. By all accounts, he was a very popular and generous person who commanded the respect of everyone. He also founded a college in Hobart, Australia, endowed with his own private funds and established the Royal Society of Tasmania, again at his own expense.

In true British Empire tradition, Secretary Barrow continued to seek the elusive Northwest Passage and set about organizing a grand expedition to achieve this goal in 1845. Upon his return to England, Sir John Franklin learned of the polar expedition and that the admiralty still had great confidence in him. This was somewhat surprising, since he was now close to sixty years old. Without any hesitation, he accepted their invitation to lead this demanding challenge.

Franklin's fame and prestige attracted a throng of volunteers from all classes of society who wanted to join his expedition. Two ships, the *Terror* and the *Erebus*, were specially outfitted to withstand the rigors of Arctic travel. No expense was to be spared and that included the food provisions. By this time, canned foods had proven to be highly acceptable to all mariners. Although they were more expensive than traditional stores, their convenience made them worth every penny.

Ever the enterprising businessman, Stephan Goldner obtained a major order to supply the canned foods for the Franklin expedition. Included in the order were 31,000 pounds of meat, 5,500 pounds of vegetables, and 22,000 pints of soup. Two weeks before the planned departure of the expedition, the superintendent of provisions reported that Goldner had supplied only 10 percent of the contracted amount. Under tremendous pressure, Goldner promised three days later that all the meat would be ready by May 12 and the soup by May 15. More important, he asked to be allowed to supply the soup in larger canisters than originally agreed in order to speed up his deliveries (since he would have to construct fewer cans). He received approval for this. On May 15, Goldner again scribbled a note to the admiralty, saying that there would be a slight delay in the soup delivery. Two days before departure, the products finally arrived.

On May 19, 1845, outfitted with a five-year supply of food provisions, Franklin triumphantly sailed down the Thames River as head of the biggest, best-equipped, and most costly naval expedition ever mounted. In the name of Queen and Country, he was all set to make history.

History was made, but, sadly, it was not that which was intended. The two ships, *Erebus* and *Terror*, were last sighted on July 26, 1845, by British whalers who were plying the seas north of Baffin Island. No other sighting was ever made, nor a word heard from the expedition—a crushing blow to the pride of the empire. Two years later, out of great concern for the fate of the 128 officers and men, a series of search parties was sent out. For a number of years, they searched in vain.

By 1847 canned preserves had become a standard ration in the British navy, and Goldner profited handsomely by putting both his factories to work supplying products. However, a significant portion of his sales to the navy seemed to spoil after relatively short periods.

In 1849 the number of negative reports regarding faulty cans and spoiled products coming in from the Naval Supply Yards became too great to ignore. A year later, one of these yards condemned more than one hundred thousand pounds of Goldner's meat products. Goldner himself came under immediate suspicion, particularly his operation in Romania.

Not only was Goldner refused further orders from the navy, but the outrage caused by such large product condemnations led to demands for an official investigation. A government select committee was established to look into the matter. Goldner testified that he felt the problems originated in the demand for larger-sized tins (even though it was he who made the request to produce them for the Franklin expedition, in order to save time and expense). He felt that it was much more difficult to expel the oxygen from these large containers compared to the smaller canisters.

The committee investigation demonstrated a clear correlation between the general introduction of large containers (nine to thirty-two pounds) in 1849 and the subsequent increase in rates of spoilage. They noted that the six-pound or smaller cans had hardly any problems. The committee issued its report in 1852, recommending that the maximum size can be six pounds and that the navy set up its own cannery at the Deptford Supply Yard.

In August 1850, the British ship *Assistance*, captained by Erasmus Ommanney, found the first traces of the Franklin expedition at Cape Riley on Devon Island. A few days later, three graves were found side by side in the shallow permafrost on nearby Beechy Island. The headstones indicated that the sailors died during the first winter of the expedition—a sure sign of major problems. An equally disturbing sign of problems was the stacks of abandoned tinned foods also found on Beechy Island. The only reason they would have been abandoned so early was that they were considered to be spoiled. Analysis showed that the cans did indeed contain rotten meat. Ommanney asserted that the cans were filled with "putrid abominations," concluding that the long-term supply of the expedition's provisions had been critically compromised.

In 1854, explorer John Rae returned from the search for Franklin with the sad news that the expedition survivors had abandoned the ice-locked ships and attempted to trek across the frozen tundra. He based his comments on the reports of Inuit hunters who had seen the remains of an estimated forty sailors. Rae went on to say that it was evident the sailors had been forced to resort to cannibalism in order to survive. "From the mutilated state of many of the bodies and the contents of the kettles, it is evident that our wretched Countrymen had been driven to the last dread alternative—cannibalism—as a means of prolonging existence." This caused a storm of protest in England, where everyone refused to believe that sailors of the Royal Navy could ever do such a thing.

In an article titled "The Lost Arctic Voyagers" published in the magazine *Household Words* on December 2, 1854, Charles Dickens maintained that there was no reason whatever to believe that any members of the expedition prolonged their existence by "the dreadful expedient of eating the bodies of their dead companions." Instead, with an implied racism that was common throughout the empire at the time, he blamed the Inuit.

> Lastly, no man can, with any show of reason, undertake to affirm that this sad remnant of Franklin's gallant band were not set upon and slain by the Esquimaux themselves. It is impossible to form an estimate of the character of any race of savages, from their deferential behavior to the white man while he is strong. The mistake has been made again and again; and the moment the white man has appeared in the new aspect of being weaker than the savage, the savage has changed and sprung upon him. . . . We believe every savage to be in his heart covetous, treacherous, and cruel.[7]

Strange words from the supposed champion of human rights.

In fact, further research proved that Rae's assessment was quite correct. In 1857, after unsuccessfully pleading with the navy and after an unsatisfactory attempt to gain the influence of politician Benjamin Disraeli to send out a last search party, Lady Jane Franklin personally paid to outfit a final expedition under Sir Francis McClintock to search for her husband. Reaching King William Island, McClintock encountered a party of Inuit with several Franklin expedition relics in their possession. They told him that they acquired the clothes and artifacts from a large shipwreck years earlier. On May 29, 1859, McClintock came across the first skeleton, still fully garbed in a steward's uniform. The notebook found beside him stated that he was Harry Peglar, petty officer of HMS *Terror*.

Another search party found the only written record of the Franklin expedition, indicating that Franklin himself had died on June 11, 1847, two years after setting sail. The record also indicated that nine other officers and fifteen crewmen died as well. The two ships had been stuck in the ice since September 12, 1846, and the remainder of the party had struck out across the tundra in a desperate attempt to survive.

Further searching revealed a strange assortment of the sailors' remains. Foods such as chocolate and tea together with an enormous quantity of goods useless to their circumstances, such as books, slippers, soap, and combs were found. The additional burden these ridiculous articles would have required led the searchers to believe that the men of the expedition had gone berserk.

Upon his return, McClintock's report devastated the nation. So many lives lost. What had gone wrong? How could a superbly equipped and provisioned expedition led by a Knight of the Crown come to such a disastrous and ignominious end? Several attempts were made to find the remains of the other crew members and the wreckage of the two ships, but without any success.

A debate regarding the cause of the disaster has gone on for more than a century. The few clues available led to certain assumptions. The large store of unused cans found by Captain Ommanney combined with the charges leveled at Goldner for selling the navy substandard products led to the inescapable conclusion that a major factor contributing to the demise of the expeditioners was the state of the canned provisions. Not only was a large proportion of their food supply unavailable (a disastrous event for any Arctic exploration), but it was possible that the limited consumption of the canned goods resulted in widespread food poisoning.

A recent book by Scott Cookman suggests that the cans were contaminated with botulism and that this toxin caused the ultimate demise of the expeditioners.[8] Although this premise is theoretically possible, it is unlikely.

Botulism is a very serious illness that results in muscle paralysis. It is caused by the botulinum neurotoxin. Botulinum toxin is a byproduct of the metabolism of the microorganism *Clostridium botulinum*. A key characteristic of this organism is that it can form spores that are very resistant to extreme conditions of heat and dryness. A second, even more important characteristic is that these microorganisms live in the absence of oxygen—they are anaerobic. In fact, they will die when exposed to oxygen, which is why they form spores—in order to seal them off from the air in our atmosphere.

Clostridium spores are ubiquitous in the environment. They exist in great numbers in the soil, and we ingest them all the time. The spores do not form toxins in our digestive systems. And even when the bacterial cells "hatch" from the spores, they are not likely to produce any toxins because of our acidic gastric juices.

Botulism poisoning symptoms usually begin to appear from twelve to thirty-six hours after eating contaminated foods. They start at the top of the body and work their way down toward the feet (this is called descending paralysis). The first symptoms are blurred or double vision and dizziness, followed by difficulty in swallowing and speaking. The muscles become weak, and breathing becomes difficult because the diaphragm can no longer drive the lungs to fill with air. Once this happens, death proceeds very quickly.

Because they were considered to be superior to other provisions, canned products would have been consumed throughout the voyage from England to the Arctic. If that was the case, there should have been some record or note describing the death of sailors or officers during the first leg of the voyage. No evidence of any kind indicates that this occurred.

The select committee report stated that the contents of Goldner's canned goods putrefied because not all of the air had been eliminated. Of course, the presence of any air would not have allowed the *Clostridium* bacteria to survive and produce toxin.

Finally, death from botulism is a rapid and dramatic process that can affect a great many people because of the potency of the toxin. Apart from the fact that the expedition had unloaded their store of canned goods on Beechy Island, the limited number of deaths was the only indication that something was wrong—not what one might expect from a large crew suffering from a botulism outbreak.

Taken in total, there is far more evidence against botulism as the cause of the disaster than for it. However, the men did unload a great deal of canned food products on Beechy Island and carried with them a large number of items that were totally useless. Had they really gone out of their minds? Quite possibly!

In 1981 Owen Beattie, an anthropologist at the University of Alberta, found the skulls and bones of two expedition crewmen and analyzed them. The results showed very high levels of lead. Three years later, he collected additional material for analysis from the body of a crewman who had been well preserved in the permafrost. The hair samples (which can provide an excellent indication of what was consumed during the previous few months) showed lead levels that were 120 times above normal.[9]

Beattie also examined the tin cans that were found on Beechy Island. He noticed that the inside seams had large gobs of solder protruding—an indication of sloppy construction. The solder originally used to seal can seams contained more than 50 percent lead. When the food made contact with lead, the possibility of lead contamination increased. This increase would be dramatic if the food was acidic enough to actively leach the lead out of the solder—a common occurrence in spoiled products.

The expedition spent its first winter (1845) on Beechy Island. The second winter (1846) was spent on the northwest coast of King William Island. Unfortunately, the winter was so severe that the ice failed to melt in 1847 and the ships were forced to spend another winter locked in.

By 1848 the crew had gone without fresh food for three years. Twenty-four of the crew had died, and the remaining 105 men decided to abandon their vessels and take their chances on an overland trek. The cumulative effects of bad weather, a lack of satisfactory provisions, and an overextended period of inadequate nutrition resulted in a crew that was totally unable to deal with the severe challenges of the Arctic. There is little doubt that conditions such as scurvy, pneumonia, and tuberculosis also ravaged the men.

Heavy-metal poisoning, such as from lead, routinely results in symptoms of mental instability and can lead to lapses in judgment (the Roman emperors are a prime example of this). Beattie's excellent analysis showed that the lead solder in the cans and the lead content of the hair samples contained the very same isotope—proof that the lead poisoning the men suffered came from the cans made by Goldner.

While there is little doubt that several factors played a hand in the challenges faced by the Franklin expedition, there can be little doubt that food poisoning and Goldner's canned products contributed in large part to the ultimate demise of one of history's great expeditions. Such are the risks that accompanied the exploration of new frontiers.

During the twentieth century, there were several successful voyages through the Northwest Passage. However, to this day, a commercially viable shipping route has not been established. Unfortunately, the impact of global warming upon the Arctic waters may soon make the Northwest Passage a practical reality.

EVENT 12. THE STAFF OF LIFE OR DEATH? HONG KONG'S ESING BAKERY

> Oh! God! that bread should be so dear,
> And flesh and blood so cheap!
>
> Thomas Hood (1799–1845),
> British poet and humorist

On August 8, 2001, *China's Peoples Daily* reported that more than 120 people in Ningxiang who ate noodles at sixteen different restaurants became ill and were hospitalized. As it turned out, the noodles were contaminated with rat poison. The incident was considered to be an act of sabotage by two men angry at the noodle factory's owners because of an ongoing business feud.

A year later, on September 14, 2002, the Chinese government reported that a large number of people became violently ill after buying food from the Zhengwu Pastry Bar in Tangshan, a suburb of Nanjing. The products were sesame cakes, fried dough sticks, and other types of glutinous rice snacks. The Official China News Agency would only admit to "a number of deaths." The owner of the shop was immediately detained.

However, within a short time, Mr. Chen, age thirty-two, who ran a snack bar in competition with the Zhengwu Pastry Bar, was arrested and quickly brought to trial. According to the court, he deliberately poisoned the products because he was jealous of the Zhengwu Pastry Bar's success. Chen admitted to putting a large amount of a powerful rat poison into his rival's raw pastry materials on September 13. More than three hundred people who had breakfast there the next day became ill, and forty-two eventually died.

In order to suppress the bad publicity and to bring the perpetrator to swift justice, the Intermediate People's Court of Nanjing found Chen guilty and immediately sentenced him to death on September 30, 2002.

Just two months later, a food-poisoning incident in a kindergarten in Wuzhou in South China's Guangdong Province put seventy children and two teachers in the hospital. The *Southern City Post* said that just after noon on November 25, 2002, most of the children in the kindergarten began to vomit and go into convulsions after eating lunch. According to the initial diagnosis, the children had eaten food contaminated with rat poison.

On October 23, 2003, it was reported that ten people died after rat poison was deliberately put into food for guests at a rural funeral in Lichuan City in central China's Hubei Province. Police investigations and hospital tests showed that the victims, ten of whom died on the spot and twenty-three who were hospitalized, had consumed a rat poison that was banned from production or sale in China. Chen Xiaomei, the widow of the deceased, was detained by the police for planning a mass poisoning at the funeral banquet in honor of her husband. It turns out that there was a long-standing feud among the family about issues such as division of property, support of the elderly parents, and various problems with the in-laws.

On July 1, 2005, *Independent Online* reported that China's capital, Beijing, sounded an alarm over an explosion in its rat population, voicing fears that rats could pose a health risk during the 2008 Olympics. (I suspect the cause was the shortage of rat poison resulting from its misappropriation for other nefarious uses.)

The deliberate poisoning of food is not a new phenomenon, particularly in China. In fact, one of the largest mass-poisoning incidents in recent history—nothing less than the attempted murder of an entire ethnic community—occurred in Hong Kong during the height of the second Sino-British Opium War, a little over a century ago.

The twentieth century may have belonged to America, but the nineteenth century was definitely the property of Merry Olde England. The two mottoes "Britannia rules the waves" and "the sun never sets on the British Empire" were not idle clichés, they were political realities. Like all other empires, the British Empire was not the product of the spontaneous acceptance of Britain's cultural values and way of life. Who would voluntarily eat "toad in the hole" (Yorkshire pudding stuffed with a pork sausage) or "bubble and squeak" (a mushy dish of cabbage, potatoes, and carrots fried in lard)? No, the empire was the product of a military might whose singular goal was to hijack the economies and natural endowments of its colonies in order to bolster its own wealth.

Throughout the eighteenth and nineteenth centuries, all of Europe—the British in particular—was enthralled with everything Oriental. Dutch, Portuguese, and British traders amassed incredible wealth by delivering exotic Asian goods to markets fascinated with everything coming out of the Far East. There was a great demand for silks, tea, and ceramics, as well as the intricate handicrafts and fireworks the Chinese produced. China was making a fortune in international trade, much as it does today, but without the help of Wal-Mart.

The problem was that the Manchu leaders of the Qing dynasty did not particularly like Westerners and were suspicious of their influence on China's people and their way of life. Imperial China's leaders were fully aware of the growth of British colonialism throughout Asia and did not want to be subject to it, nor did they relish buying English goods that were inevitably foisted upon the colonists. As a result, Chinese products were sent out of the country, but no British products or traders were allowed into China. To enforce the sanction on foreign imports, China demanded silver as the exclusive form of payment for all its exports.

British trade with China was in the hands of the one company to which parliament had granted an exclusive commercial monopoly, the venerable British East India Company. When it was originally founded and chartered by Queen Elizabeth I in 1600, the company was called the Governor and Company of Merchants of London Trading into the East Indies. It was an enterprise of London businessmen who joined together to import spices from South Asia. Prior to that time, the spice trade with the East Indies relied exclusively upon land routes across the Middle East and Asia, but through the expert seamanship of the Portuguese, Europeans began to import products directly and were able to cut out all the intermediaries. Initially, it was the Spanish and the Portuguese who held a monopoly over the East Indian spice trade until the destruction of the Spanish Armada in 1588. This permitted the British and the Dutch to enter into this lucrative enterprise.

Despite its enormous trading power and influence, the British East India Company fell upon difficult times with China because of the great imbalance of trade and, more particularly, because of China's demand for silver in exchange for all its goods. The company then hit upon the idea of exchanging opium, grown in another of Britain's colonies, India, for the valuable Chinese goods. The managers of the British East India Company worked out a cunning scheme of selling licenses to private traders to sell opium to the Chinese in exchange for silver. This silver was then cashed in for letters of credit, and the British East India Company used the silver to finance the purchase of Chinese goods destined for England. No wonder Britannia ruled the waves.

Once exposed to opium, China rapidly developed the habit. Within a relatively short period of time, the balance of trade shifted against the Chinese. The country was also starting to experience the ravages of opium smoking. The Qing government tried to impose a ban on opium importation in 1800, but it met with little success. This was followed thirteen years later with an outright ban on the use of opium, but by then it was too late. Opium addiction was widespread, and the profits from that trade enticed a limitless supply of smugglers willing to risk the consequences of defying the law—not too great in a government riddled with corruption.

When Britain abolished the British East India Company's monopoly in 1834, it opened up a bonanza in the opium trading business. A few years later, the imperial commissioner in Canton, Lin Tse Hsu, was given the task of ending the trade in opium. He sent a well-publicized letter to Queen Victoria requesting that Britain cease all opium trade with China. He stressed that because opium trade and consumption was illegal in Britain and because of the devastation caused, it should never be exported to other countries. The British, however, were not in a mood to listen to logic or fair play, because they were making so much money. Lin's plea fell on deaf ears.

In 1839, in a desperate attempt to curb the opium trade, Lin then threatened to cut off all trade with the British and to expel its citizens and traders from Canton and Macao. Shortly thereafter, he followed through with his threat. In the process of expelling the traders, he forced them to hand over all their supplies of opium and then ordered it burned in public. Lin thought that would be the end of it. But the unyielding British had other plans. Thus began the first Opium War in 1839.

Although Hong Kong was inhabited as far back as the Stone Age, it was never considered to be important by the Chinese emperors. It was a sleepy little island of farmers and fishermen. However, its well-sheltered deepwater harbor made it a haven for pirates of all kinds. And it was for that geographical asset that the British decided to steal it.

The Opium War was little more than a series of sporadic bombardments and raids on Chinese coastal settlements by the British. It escalated dramatically when a contingent of fourteen thousand Royal Marines attacked Hong Kong on January 26, 1841. Despite fierce resistance by the local inhabitants, the marines prevailed and claimed the island as a British possession. It formally became a colony of Britain in 1842 as part of the Treaty of Nanking, the agreement to end the first Opium War. The treaty was overwhelmingly in Britain's favor and was a great humiliation to the Chinese.

The opium trade continued to flourish with Hong Kong as its commercial base. The relationships between the Chinese and the British continued to be strained—no surprise if one considers how one-sided the

Treaty of Nanking was. Nonetheless, British traders were also unhappy because the Chinese weren't consuming opium fast enough for them.

All this discontent ignited a second Opium War that began in 1856. It started when a small ship called the *Arrow*, owned by a Chinese resident of Hong Kong, was boarded by Chinese officials in search of evidence of smuggling and piracy. The problem was that the ship was temporarily registered with the British in Hong Kong and was flying a British flag. The Chinese officials boarded the ship without asking Britain's permission as was stipulated by the Treaty of Nanking (in fact, it was a perfectly legal move, since the temporary registration had by that time expired). To make matters worse, the Chinese officials hauled down the British flag.

Whether or not the British took the trouble to check that the British registration had expired is still a matter of conjecture. In a manner fully consistent with their arrogant and belligerent foreign policy, the British immediately used the incident as a convenient excuse to precipitate military action to force the Chinese to take more goods in trade, especially opium. This period of military skirmishes constituted the second Opium War.

It was against this explosive backdrop of political upheaval, harsh military domination, and national humiliation that a plot was hatched to strike back at the British through an act of civilian terrorism. The goal of this plan was ambitious—nothing less than the murder of all the Westerners living in Hong Kong!

The idea behind the scheme was simple. Asians ate rice while Westerners ate bread. Resorting to a time-honored method of murder common throughout China, the perpetrators decided to use poison—they laced Hong Kong's bread supply with arsenic. Most of the foreigners in the British colony bought their bread from the Esing Bakery in the Spring Gardens district of Hong Kong, and that was where the poisoning originated.

On the morning of January 15, 1857, hundreds of Hong Kong's foreign residents were stricken with acute arsenic poisoning. Not only were Europeans and Americans affected but the community of Indian ɔrtunately, for Cheung's sake, the prosecutor was Attorney General ɦomas Chisholm Anstey, known as one of the greatest blowhards in ɛ entire British Empire. Since no one had actually died by the time ɾ the trial and because Cheung's own children had also been poisoned . the incident, the tide of sympathy turned his way. Anstey countered ı open court with "Better to hang the wrong man, than confess that ɾitish sagacity and activity have failed to discover the real criminals." ɦe judge rebuked Anstey for that comment, and eventually the court ɔund Cheung not guilty by a five-to-one majority.

Even though he was found innocent of the charges, Cheung was ɛported and eventually settled in Vietnam, where he became a cele-ɾated and wealthy businessman, highly honored by the French colo-ɭalists.[13] Anstey returned to Britain in 1861 and, in keeping with his yle, aired his grievances regarding the governance of Hong Kong in 116-page letter to the *Times*—the longest letter ever sent to that ɛwspaper.

Eventually it was deduced that two of Cheung's foremen were the ɔtual perpetrators, but they had long since made their successful ɔcape back to mainland China.

The Esing Bakery incident is an excellent example of how, under ɛrtain conditions, a particular community can be specifically and suc-ɛssfully targeted for terrorist action through food poisoning.

ɪOTES

1. E. Hesketh, *J. & E. Hall Ltd. 1785–1935* (Glasgow: Glasgow Uni-ɛrsity Press, 1935).

2. *Historic Tinned Foods Publication # 85*, International Tin Research ɪd Development Council (Middlesex, England: Greenfield, 1939).

3. Sir John Pringle, "A Discourse upon Some Late Improvements of ɛe Means for Preserving the Health of Mariners (1776)," in *Historic Tinned ɔods, Publication #85.*

4. J. Cutbush, *Lecture on the Adulteration of Foods and Culinary Poi-ɔns* (Newburgh, NY: W. M. Gazlay, 1823).

Jews who made up a large part of the civil service was
well. They were the first to be hit because they arose
breakfast earlier than the rest of the city. In fact, the
calamity in the Indian community quickly served a
others and limited the scope of the incident.[10]

The owner of the Esing Bakery was Cheung A
morning of the poisoning incident, Cheung and his fan
steamer *Shamrock*, which was headed for Macao. Bec
of poisoning was quickly determined to be the bread
Bakery, suspicion immediately fell upon Cheung. As th
community in Hong Kong was in an uproar, the police
react. A private citizen, W. H. Robinet, took it upon h
private steamer, the *Spark*, and pursue the *Shamrock* to

As it happened, the *Shamrock* purchased its brea
the Esing Bakery, and during the five-hour trip to Mac
sengers who ate the bread got violently ill. The cap
Cheung the baker and his family among the passengers
detain them pending news from the authorities in H
Spark soon arrived, and at Robinet's request, Cheung
the Portuguese authorities and sent back to Hong Kon

Fortunately, in their zeal to kill as many people as p
petrators had used far too much arsenic so that it ac
emetic, causing everyone to vomit up most of the mat
Hong Kong's surgeon general ordered additional eme
and egg white to be administered, hence the damage was

In all the confusion, no one took the trouble to
John Bowring on the morning of the incident until his
ished consuming their morning bread. He wrote, "It l
some days in racking headaches, pains to the limb
Sadly, his wife, Lady Bowring, never fully recovered
that year. Two American captains of merchant ships a
within a year of the incident.[12]

Cheung and several supposed accomplices were br
charges of "administering poison with the intent to ki

Jews who made up a large part of the civil service was struck down as well. They were the first to be hit because they arose and took their breakfast earlier than the rest of the city. In fact, the early morning calamity in the Indian community quickly served as a warning to others and limited the scope of the incident.[10]

The owner of the Esing Bakery was Cheung Ah-Lum. On the morning of the poisoning incident, Cheung and his family boarded the steamer *Shamrock*, which was headed for Macao. Because the source of poisoning was quickly determined to be the bread from the Esing Bakery, suspicion immediately fell upon Cheung. As the entire foreign community in Hong Kong was in an uproar, the police had no time to react. A private citizen, W. H. Robinet, took it upon himself to hire a private steamer, the *Spark*, and pursue the *Shamrock* to Macao.

As it happened, the *Shamrock* purchased its bread supplies from the Esing Bakery, and during the five-hour trip to Macao, several passengers who ate the bread got violently ill. The captain recognized Cheung the baker and his family among the passengers and decided to detain them pending news from the authorities in Hong Kong. The *Spark* soon arrived, and at Robinet's request, Cheung was arrested by the Portuguese authorities and sent back to Hong Kong in chains.[11]

Fortunately, in their zeal to kill as many people as possible, the perpetrators had used far too much arsenic so that it acted more as an emetic, causing everyone to vomit up most of the material consumed. Hong Kong's surgeon general ordered additional emetics of mustard and egg white to be administered, hence the damage was greatly limited.

In all the confusion, no one took the trouble to warn Governor John Bowring on the morning of the incident until his family had finished consuming their morning bread. He wrote, "It left its effect for some days in racking headaches, pains to the limbs and bowels." Sadly, his wife, Lady Bowring, never fully recovered and died later that year. Two American captains of merchant ships also succumbed within a year of the incident.[12]

Cheung and several supposed accomplices were brought to trial on charges of "administering poison with the intent to kill and murder."

Fortunately, for Cheung's sake, the prosecutor was Attorney General Thomas Chisholm Anstey, known as one of the greatest blowhards in the entire British Empire. Since no one had actually died by the time of the trial and because Cheung's own children had also been poisoned in the incident, the tide of sympathy turned his way. Anstey countered in open court with "Better to hang the wrong man, than confess that British sagacity and activity have failed to discover the real criminals." The judge rebuked Anstey for that comment, and eventually the court found Cheung not guilty by a five-to-one majority.

Even though he was found innocent of the charges, Cheung was deported and eventually settled in Vietnam, where he became a celebrated and wealthy businessman, highly honored by the French colonialists.[13] Anstey returned to Britain in 1861 and, in keeping with his style, aired his grievances regarding the governance of Hong Kong in a 116-page letter to the *Times*—the longest letter ever sent to that newspaper.

Eventually it was deduced that two of Cheung's foremen were the actual perpetrators, but they had long since made their successful escape back to mainland China.

The Esing Bakery incident is an excellent example of how, under certain conditions, a particular community can be specifically and successfully targeted for terrorist action through food poisoning.

NOTES

1. E. Hesketh, *J. & E. Hall Ltd. 1785–1935* (Glasgow: Glasgow University Press, 1935).

2. *Historic Tinned Foods Publication # 85*, International Tin Research and Development Council (Middlesex, England: Greenfield, 1939).

3. Sir John Pringle, "A Discourse upon Some Late Improvements of the Means for Preserving the Health of Mariners (1776)," in *Historic Tinned Foods, Publication #85*.

4. J. Cutbush, *Lecture on the Adulteration of Foods and Culinary Poisons* (Newburgh, NY: W. M. Gazlay, 1823).

5. "Meriwether Lewis Goes Shopping," *Calendar Features April 2004 Feature*, National Archives, http://www.archives.gov/calendar/features /2004/04.html (accessed July 28, 2005).

6. Otto von Kotzebue, *A Voyage of Discovery, into the South Sea and Beering's Straits, for the Purpose of Exploring a North-East Passage, undertaken in the Years 1815–1818, in the Ship Rurick* (London: Longman, Hurst, Rees, Orme and Brown, 1821).

7. Charles Dickens, "The Lost Arctic Voyagers," *Household Words* (December 2 and 9, 1854).

8. S. Cookman, *Ice Blink: The Tragic Fate of Sir John Franklin's Lost Polar Expedition* (New York: John Wiley and Sons, 2000).

9. Z. B. Horowitz, "Polar Poisons: Did Botulism Doom the Franklin Expedition?" *Journal of Toxicology—Clinical Toxicology* 41, no. 6 (2003): 841–47.

10. J. P. Griffen, "Famous Names: The Esing Bakery, Hong Kong," *Adverse Drug Reactions and Toxicolical Reviews* 16, no. 2 (1997): 79–81.

11. A. F. Heard, "Poisoning by Wholesale: A Reminiscence of China Life, with an Introduction by Robert M. Gray," in *Augustine Heard and Company, 1858–1862: American Merchants in China*, by S. C. Lockwood, Harvard East Asian Monographs 37 (1971), http://www-ee.stanford.edu/~gray/ poisoning.pdf (accessed July 28, 2005).

12. L. and M. Ride, *East India Company Cemetery*, ed. B. Mellor (Hong Kong: Hong Kong University Press, 1996).

13. Choi Chi-cheung, "Cheung Ah-Lum, A Biographical Note," *Journal of the Royal Asiatic Society Hong Kong Branch* 24 (1984): 282–85.

CHAPTER 6
MODERN TIMES
(1900 CE–Present Day)

Based on the understanding of food and beverage spoilage gained in the latter half of the nineteenth century, an explosion of technological improvements set the stage for a revolution in the production and processing that redefined the foods we eat and the manner in which we consume them. The twentieth century started with the average consumer eating home-cooked fresh meals that relied heavily on locally available products such as meat, potatoes, dairy, and seasonable vegetables. Rapid advances in food-preservation technology made a wide variety of foods much more convenient and available throughout the year. Consumer acceptance of these products allowed very large quantities to be processed during a single growing season, which in turn encouraged mass production of agricultural products because of the obvious economies based on volume. Likewise, the marketing of foods was carried out in much larger retail outlets that offered consumers convenience because of the great variety of goods one could buy at a single location.

By processing more and more foods and beverages in large production facilities, products became cheaper and more convenient. As processed foods proliferated, home cooking declined. The responsibility for safe foods passed from the homemaker to the commercial processor. Because of the shameful and corrupt behavior of several companies, however, new food-safety legislation was promulgated and mechanisms were developed to enforce the new laws. Although this was a great leap forward, major scandals continued to occur.

SINCLAIR'S *JUNGLE* AND THE WILEY FDA

The United States is a nation of laws: badly written and randomly enforced.

Frank Zappa, US musician and songwriter (1940–1993)

It seems that we never tire of saying that America is a land of laws— a land where people can live with the confidence of not having to rely on the trust between individuals. Unfortunately, this notion is understandable because our daily experiences reflect the antagonistic relationship between individuals even though most of us share common values. This antagonism is most obvious in a buyer-and-seller relationship in which each individual tries to end up with the greater advantage.

Rather than relying on trust and goodwill, most nations have opted to enact laws and standards that provide a reliable and predictable system for commercial exchanges. This system of laws and standards has been a common feature of the civilized landscape for thousands of years. Some of the earliest historical records reveal that government authorities were concerned with creating laws to protect consumers from dishonest food merchants. Assyrian tablets describe the methods to be used to establish correct weights and measures in the sale of food grains, and Egyptian papyrus scrolls stipulate the labeling that had to be applied to certain foods. Strict regulations and standards for temple sacrifices are liberally scattered throughout the Bible. The Athenians inspected their wines for purity, and the neighboring Romans developed state-organized systems to protect consumers from food fraud.

Medieval European countries instituted laws that established the quality of eggs, cheese, bread, beer, and sausages.

Thus, the concept of being a land of laws is not a new one.

The main reason that food and beverage standards have been a preoccupation for so long is because it is so easy to cheat a customer when making these products. Consider bread. Wheat flour, the main component in bread, is a product of milled wheat. Wheat is simply a seed composed of an outside layer of bran, a starchy main body (called the endosperm), and a small oil-rich section called the germ. The lightest and so-called finest bread is made from the purified endosperm because it is white and contains chiefly starch and gluten. Gluten is a unique protein that is very elastic when wet and can trap all the little bubbles formed from yeast fermentation. Aside from being elastic, gluten is what is called a thermosetting protein, which means that after baking, the spongy structure turns solid. This results in a light white bread containing thousands of tiny holes (formerly yeast gas bubbles).

By far the most valuable and expensive part of wheat flour has traditionally been the purified endosperm. The bran and germ were considered to be by-products. Of course, this valuation has little to do with nutrition—it merely reflects the requirements of the market at a specific time and place. These days, bran and germ have much greater value because whole-wheat and multigrain products are "in" as a result of nutritional concerns.

When white flour was all the rage, unscrupulous millers and merchants would often augment their profits by adding chalk (soft, porous limestone) or white ash to the final product. It is amazing how forgiving wheat gluten proteins can be, because the adding of up to 10 to 15 percent of light-colored foreign material to flour could easily go unnoticed in the final product.

Inevitably, such adulterations became uncovered, and laws or standards were issued to make it a crime to misrepresent the products sold in any commercial transaction.

The First Assize of Bread directed at the Bakers of the City of York

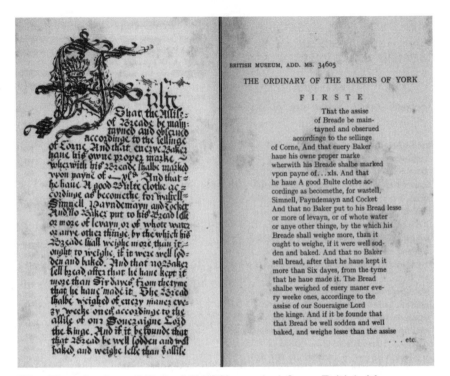

The First Assize of Bread (1589), copied from British Museum Manuscript #34605.

in England was issued in the year 1589, over four hundred years ago. It stated that bread had to have the name of the baker stamped on it and that the wheat used should be properly sieved through a standardized bolting (sifting) cloth. Bread was also to have the proper weight of ingredients and was to be sold before the end of its six-day shelf life— all in all, a fairly complete standard.

Despite the laws and penalties against food and beverage adulteration, the practice continued throughout history. An excellent treatise on the subject was written by Frederick Accum. Accum was a German chemist who immigrated to London in 1793 to work as a chemical analyst and teacher. Accum became aware of the problem of food adulteration through his analytical work and, in 1820, published *A Treatise on*

Adulterations of Food and Culinary Poisons in order to expose the widespread extent of the dismal practice. The first edition sold out quickly, and a US edition was published in Philadelphia the same year. Accum was passionate about the issue and regarded the adulteration of food and drink as a criminal offense. On page 22, he states: "The man who robs a fellow subject of a few shillings on the high-way, is sentenced to death; while he who distributes a slow poison to a whole community, escapes unpunished."[1]

Accum described the adulteration of beer with ferrous sulphate, extracts of *Cocculus indicus* (a narcotic stimulant), quassia (a bitter bark extract used as an insecticide), and liquorice juice to impart bitterness to the brew without the expense of using natural hops. He showed how red wine was diluted with the juice of bilberries or elderberries and how cream could be cheapened with starch pastes. He considered the use of artificial colors (often containing lead, copper, or mercury salts) to mislead the public into buying low-quality jams, jellies, and sweets to be the most reprehensible practice, because children were among the main consumers. He went as far as publishing the names of manufacturers and traders convicted of adulterating food and drink with poisonous additives. As a result, he made himself some very powerful enemies.

Accum was secretly observed and was eventually accused of mutilating some books in the library of the Royal Institution. His premises were searched, and pages torn out of books were found, though it was never established whether they were from his own book collection or from that of the Royal Institution. He was charged and appeared before the court. Because he felt he was publicly disgraced, he immediately fled back to Germany when released on bail. As a result, his extraordinary and accurate portrayal of illegitimate food practices was largely forgotten, and the industry went merrily back to its old practices.

The situation was not very different in the United States. Until the beginning of the twentieth century, very little national legislation existed, and individual states administered control over the trade in food and beverages. This resulted in a great deal of inconsistency in

A

TREATISE

ON

ADULTERATIONS OF FOOD,

AND CULINARY POISONS.

EXHIBITING

The Fraudulent Sophistications of

BREAD, BEER, WINE, SPIRITOUS LIQUORS,
TEA, COFFEE, CREAM, CONFECTIONERY,
VINEGAR, MUSTARD, PEPPER, CHEESE,
OLIVE OIL, PICKLES,
AND OTHER ARTICLES EMPLOYED IN DOMESTIC ECONOMY.

AND

METHODS OF DETECTING THEM.

———

By Fredrick Accum,

OPERATIVE CHEMIST, AND MEMBER OF THE PRINCIPAL
ACADEMIES AND SOCIETIES OF ARTS AND SCIENCES
IN EUROPE.

———

Philadelphia:

PRINTED AND PUBLISHED BY AB'M SMALL.

1820.

Frontispiece from Fredrick Accum, *A Treatise on Adulterations of Food and Culinary Poisons* (Philadelphia: Abraham Small, 1820).

the quality of goods from one state to another. It also forced manufacturers to set different standards for the different states.

By the late nineteenth century, adulteration remained a common practice for many food and beverage manufacturers. In order to curb this practice of deceiving consumers, a growing pure-foods movement developed in the United States during the 1870s. The movement was instigated by several of the large food companies who felt that the public's confidence in foods was being eroded by the many unscrupulous fly-by-night operators who cobbled together products from cheap ingredients and adulterants and pawned them off as high-quality goods.

Advances in food chemistry also served as motivation for food manufacturers to push for national pure-food legislation. The discovery that glucose, prepared by the acid hydrolysis of cornstarch, could serve as a cheap replacement for sugar and that oleomargarine—prepared from almost any source of animal, fish, or vegetable fat—could substitute for much more expensive butter sent shock waves through the industry. It was clearly in the commercial interests of traditional food manufacturers to push for a law that would distinguish between traditional ingredients and their chemically modified replacements.

In 1883 Dr. Harvey W. Wiley, professor of chemistry at Purdue University, became the chief chemist in the department of agriculture's division of chemistry. In this position, Wiley ushered in a new era. The division had mainly focused on analyzing soils and fertilizers; now the attention shifted to the definition and labeling of foods and beverages. Products that did not fall into the standards set were considered to be adulterated.

Adulteration does not necessarily mean that a product is physiologically harmful, it means that it does not conform to a preestablished standard. One could easily concoct an imitation strawberry jam from sugar, glucose, pectin, gelatin, alfalfa seed, and artificial color and flavor. The product may not be harmful, but it is not what consumers expect strawberry jam to be. What if the product contained 90 percent real jam and 10 percent artificial jam? Again, even though an expert may have trouble telling the difference between the two, it would be still considered adulterated, and rightly so. If the price were a dollar a jar, the consumer couldn't get away with paying ninety genuine cents and ten cents of Monopoly money!

The major impact of standards on the food industry is on the commercial bottom line. Thus, it is little wonder that manufacturers made such an effort to push for standards and labeling that favored their particular products' processes.

Corn glucose manufacturers wanted their products to be called corn syrup, so that they could compete more effectively with products such as genuine maple syrup and honey. A description of the process used to produce glucose and fructose from cornstarch would take several pages of sophisticated chemistry and engineering. But, in short, they differ greatly. Simply calling the product corn syrup would immediately allay all concerns the consumer might have with the product. The name would connote maple syrup, the evaporated sap from maple trees, or even honey, the flower nectar that is evaporated by the fanning of bees' wings. Selling their product as syrup brought a tremendous commercial advantage to the acid hydrolyzers of cornstarch!

Because there was so much money involved in the food and beverage business, and because of the promulgation of laws and standards not to its liking, the industry started to play hardball. In addition to peddling influence, manufacturers resorted to character assassination. It was every bit as vicious then as it is today.

But Wiley was fully up to the task of managing the division of chemistry. He was bold, opinionated, egotistical, and driven—precisely the mix of characteristics required to take on the wildly competing interests trying to steer the direction of food and drug legislation.

Initially, he was disturbed by commercial fraud such as rectified alcohol blends being sold as authentic straight whiskey. In time, however, he became genuinely concerned with the threats to health posed by the various additives on foods. He intuitively believed that most processed foods should be manufactured without the use of additives. His opinion was largely subjective because he did not have any definitive proof that additives were harmful. In order to support his views,

Wiley instituted a program whose fame and notoriety has survived to this day—the Poison Squad.

Beginning in 1902 and lasting until 1907, Wiley instituted a series of experiments to determine the influence of preservatives and coloring materials on health and digestion. In the basement of the Agriculture Department's former Bureau of Chemistry, located at the west end of the Mall on Independence Avenue, in Washington, DC, twelve healthy young men sat down to eat foods laced with various chemical additives.

They tested seven different substances, namely, boric acid and borax, salicylic acid and salicylates, benzoic acid and benzoates, sulfur dioxide and sulfites, formaldehyde, copper sulfate and saltpeter (potassium and sodium nitrites). The object of these experiments was to see if the preservatives and coloring materials added to foods would affect the health and digestion of these young men. Wiley considered young men more resistant to the effects of these potential toxins and would thus serve as a bellwether for the rest of the population at minimal risk to themselves.

Having first received authority from Congress to proceed, Wiley set up a small kitchen and dining room in the basement of the bureau and issued a call for volunteers from his staff to join in the experiment. He had no trouble finding twelve healthy young men who volunteered their services and took an oath to obey all the rules and regulations prescribed for the experiment. The minimum term of enlistment was one year.

Getting publicity for this experiment was not a problem because the story had a tremendous potential to catch the imagination of the public. One cub reporter, who actively followed the work of the group, called this band of devoted young men the "Poison Squad," and described the progress of the various experiments in a way that caught the public's imagination. This reporter, George Rothwell Brown, went on to become the celebrated author of the "Post-Scripts" in the *Washington Post*, as well as several books describing Washington politics.

Most of the resulting experimental data was published in the *Bulletins of the Bureau of Chemistry*. The publications immediately brought on protests from manufacturers who were using these materials. Kowtowing to these protests, the secretary of agriculture refused further publications, despite the fact that the results of the studies were duplicated elsewhere.

Wiley eventually stopped the experiments when some of the chemicals consumed made the diners so sick that they couldn't function. The press publicized this set of experiments, and their reports fascinated readers all over the United States. The work of the Poison Squad even made the minstrel shows. The tremendous publicity assisted Wiley in getting a congressional hearing to discuss food adulteration and the need for a pure-food law.

In retrospect, it is very doubtful if the work carried out by Wiley with the Poison Squad would be permitted today. From purely a scientific point of view, the experience left a great deal to be desired. But the Poison Squad did not leave an indelible mark on the history of food regulation because of its scientific significance. What made the Poison Squad such a success was its ability to capture and hold the attention of the public on the issue of food additives.

Wiley and the Poison Squad made consumers sit up and question whether the foods they routinely purchased and ate were poisoning them. It also encouraged consumers to believe that they had a crusading knight looking out for their interests. A personality cult grew around Wiley because he did not quibble; things were right or wrong, black or white. In Wiley's campaign, there was no room for doubt.

Not surprisingly, Wiley made a growing number of adversaries. This list included manufacturers of targeted foods and additives as well as officials within government circles who feared and envied his growing influence. As a federal employee, Wiley vigorously promoted a national pure-foods law, thus alienating himself from many state regulatory officials.

Because it is so much easier dealing with one federal law than with many different state laws, those companies that traded nationally were in favor of the Pure Food and Drug Act. Another factor was the ability of larger companies to develop the technology that was required to reduce or eliminate additives. However, what the smaller companies lacked in size and expertise, they made up in numbers and local political influence.

By the time it was closed down in 1907, the Poison Squad played a very significant role in paving the way for the federal regulation of foods in the United States. The Pure Food and Drug Act of 1906, also called the Wiley Act, was a direct result of this exercise.

Although the Pure Food and Drug Act had been written and proposed for legislation, competing interests delayed its passage through Congress. It is likely that the act would have remained in limbo had not two incidents influenced the public's passion and motivated President Theodore Roosevelt to come out hard in favor of the act.

The first incident was the fallout from the "embalmed meat" scandal, which occurred in the midst of the Spanish-American War (February to December 1898).

Military rations have always been considered one of the soldier's occupational hazards, but the canned meat given to the troops, who were seeking revenge for the sinking of the *Maine*, was in a class by itself. In his book *Always the Young Stranger*, Carl Sandburg described a meal aboard ship:

> A tin of "Red Horse" would be handed to one man who opened it. He put it to his nose, smelled of it, wrinkled up his face, and took a spit. The next man did the same and the next till the eight men of the mass had smelled, grimaced, and spit. Then that tin of "Red Horse" was thrown overboard for any of the fishes of the Atlantic Ocean who might like it. What we called "Red Horse" soon had all our country scandalized with its new name of "Embalmed Beef." It was embalmed! We buried it at sea because it was so duly embalmed with all the flavor of life and every suck of nourishment drawn from it though having nevertheless a putridity of odor more pungent than ever reaches the nostrils from a properly embalmed cadaver.[2]

The product in question was canned beef rations for the troops who were in transit or serving in the field. While there was no doubt that the quality of the beef used for canning was very poor, no scientific evidence was ever presented that it had been "embalmed" or treated with chemical preservatives prior to canning. All the products sent to Wiley's Bureau of Chemistry from this group were analyzed, but none exhibited evidence of chemical additives of any kind.

The notion that the canned beef was embalmed, and therefore poisonous, arose from the substantial rate of sickness that occurred among all the troops. During the Spanish-American War, only 280 American soldiers were killed in battle, while 2,630 died from other causes.[3] Major Walter Reed eventually demonstrated that this high rate of illness was a direct result of typhoid fever rather than spoiled beef. Typhoid fever was rampant in the southern staging camps of Georgia and Florida, where sanitation practices were virtually nonexistent (drinking water wells were located beside the outhouses).

Despite Walter Reed's conclusions, the myth of embalmed beef persisted for decades. As a new congressman, Fiorello LaGuardia, later to become New York City's most famous mayor, introduced a bill recommending imprisonment during peacetime and death during wartime for anyone caught selling inferior food and other goods to the armed services. As it happened, LaGuardia's father was stationed in Florida during the Spanish-American War, and his family was convinced that he had died from eating embalmed beef in 1898.[4]

In December 1897, a bill to prohibit the interstate commerce of adulterated foods and drugs was introduced, and in March 1898, the first national Pure Food and Drug Congress met in Washington, DC. The embalmed beef scandal, even though totally discredited, had a very strong influence on the promotion of pure-foods legislation proposals.

In 1904 the social activist and author Upton Sinclair spent several months visiting Chicago's infamous stockyards and meatpacking plants to gather materials for his book *The Jungle*. Although the book was a social commentary on the squalid living and onerous working conditions experienced by poor immigrants, it became best known for its graphic exposé of the horrific sanitation and production practices of most Chicago meatpacking plants.

When people learned of the garbage, filth, and tainted meat they were eating, they were outraged, none more so than President Theodore Roosevelt. He aggressively pushed Congress to enact a Pure Food Bill and on June 30, 1906, he signed the Food and Drug Act into law.

Wiley, considered the father of the Food and Drug Act, continued to butt heads against those industries and their representatives who tried to get around the law or to take advantage of its many loopholes. In fact, the original law was a rather weak instrument against fraudulent activities. For example, although the law prohibited the interstate shipment of misbranded and adulterated products, it did not require labels to state the weights or measures on a package.

Aside from false claims and sophisticated methods of adulteration, Wiley had to deal with competing commercial interests. An interesting example of this was highlighted in his book *The History of the Crime Against the Food Law*.[5]

When asked the question "What is a sardine?" the bureau prepared a decision stating that only the genuine sardine originating on the coasts of Spain, France, and the Mediterranean Islands was entitled to that name. The agriculture secretary, bowing to pressure from the commercial fish packers of Maine, referred this problem to the Fish Commission of the Department of Commerce. The Fish Commission, which had no function whatever in determining or describing misbranding, made a decision diametrically opposed to that reached by the bureau.

The name *sardine* originated from the name of the Mediterranean island Sardinia. Wiley wanted the name to signify Mediterranean pilchards. The US fishing industry wanted to trade on a well-established product name and identity. One hundred years later, there's still no definitive answer to the question "What is a sardine?" In fact, this issue surfaced again recently at the World Trade Organization, with Chile and Peru taking the Europeans to task over the official description of "sardines." The same problem exists for other foods named after a region, such as Champagne, Parma ham, Dijon mustard, or Feta cheese.

Commercial interests always dominated the interpretation and implementation of the Food and Drugs Act. This led to a great deal of bureaucratic infighting highlighted by the bitter dispute between Wiley and the secretary of agriculture. It all came to a head in 1912 when Wiley resigned. In the wake of his resignation, Wiley left behind a Bureau of Chemistry that was much larger and light-years ahead of the bureau he inherited. Wiley went on to become an outspoken advocate on consumer issues.

Shortcomings in the 1906 Food and Drugs Act permitted a great deal of fraud and adulteration to continue. Some of the products were so outrageous that they attracted the attention of the press. Books such as *Your Money's Worth*, *100,000,000 Guinea Pigs*, and the *American Chamber of Horrors* stimulated the development of a burgeoning consumer movement.[6]

A passage in *Your Money's Worth* states: "At one time 50 percent of English milk on the average was estimated to be adulterated with water. Today it is not over 10 to 15 percent. Watered milk looks bluish. To offset this, a yellow dye is introduced to restore that creamy color. When the process of sugar refining was changed, it produced a whiter sugar than people were accustomed to. To bring back to the old shade, tin chloride was added. Enameled kitchen utensils have contained poisonous lead salts. Some still contain them."[7]

This passage from *100,000,000 Guinea Pigs* gets a little more personal: "William J. A. Bailey, an ex-auto-swindler, thought he could make money by dissolving radium salts in water and selling this water to rich men to cure their ills. Bailey's radium water has sent at least two men to horrible deaths, and a similar fate may be awaiting scores or hundreds of others who drank this deadly fluid."[8]

Ruth deForest Lamb's *American Chamber of Horrors* focused on the many defective practices that were carried out despite the 1906 Food and Drugs Act:

> The old Wiley law does not prohibit deceptive containers nor slack-filled packages, and this defect has committed an anonymous amount of petty chiseling. Oatmeal, macaroni, spices and rice are particularly subject to this practice. . . . In a recent survey by State authorities in Alabama, six samples of black pepper showed a sale of container from 82 percent to as low as 43 percent of what the house-

wife might reasonably expect. Coffee and chicory compounds ranged from 67 to 80%, the average being about 70, and one sample of tea was hardly more than half full.[9]

Despite aggressive opposition by industry and advertising interests toward any revisions of the old Food and Drugs Act, organized women's clubs continued to stoke the fires and demanded that products and labeling reflect honesty and transparency. Just as Sinclair's exposure of the packinghouse conditions in Chicago captured the public's attention, another shocking incident in 1937 inflamed emotions to the extent that it was not possible to delay revising the old act. This was the 1937 Elixir Sulfanilamide incident.

> But to realize that six human beings, all of them my patients, one of them my best friend, are dead because they took medicine that I prescribed for them innocently, and to realize that that medicine which I had used for years in such cases suddenly had become a deadly poison in its newest and most modern form, as recommended by a great and reputable pharmaceutical firm in Tennessee: well, that realization has given me such days and nights of mental and spiritual agony as I did not believe a human being could undergo and survive. I have known hours when death for me would be a welcome relief from this agony. (Letter by Dr. A. S. Calhoun, October 22, 1937).[10]

This letter, written by an obviously distraught person, reflected the mood of a great many physicians. In the days before antibiotics were available, a widely prescribed medicine that held great promise to cure a range of infections had begun killing patients. In 1932 Gerhard Domagk, a chemist with the I. G. Farben Company of Germany, discovered that one of the company's red dyes was active against certain types of bacterial infections in animals. Further experiments revealed that the dye was broken down into a chemical called para-aminobenzenesulfonamide, also known as sulfanilamide. After numerous other studies, sulfanilamide was recommended by the medical establishment for use against streptococcal infections. Since sulfanilamide was first produced in 1908, it was no longer covered by any patents, so several large pharmaceutical companies began producing it.

A relatively small Tennessee-based company, S. E. Massengill, also jumped in to produce its version of the product. Although it originally began using capsules and tablets, Massengill soon concluded that there was a demand for a liquid elixir, since none was available from other sources.

The company's chief chemist was given the task of finding the best liquid to dissolve the sulfanilamide in. He settled on diethylene glycol and decided to add a raspberry extract flavoring to make it more palatable.

The 1906 Food and Drugs Act didn't require safety or toxicity studies to be carried out on new drugs. The assumption was that no company would risk selling drugs that were toxic. Massengill's new product was dubbed Elixir Sulfanilamide, even though it contained no ethanol, an ingredient normally required in all "elixirs."

Starting in early September 1937, shipments of Elixir Sulfanilamide were distributed across the United States. Within a month, reports began to flow in implicating the elixir in a number of fatalities. It did not take long to find out that diethylene glycol was the toxic ingredient. Massengill had sent out telegrams to all its customers to return the elixir, but neglected to inform them of its toxic nature. The FDA insisted on a second telegram to communicate just that warning.

The FDA then mobilized its entire field force of inspectors to ensure that all the Elixir Sulfanilamide was retrieved. This required some genuine detective work, because in certain cases, the elixir had been sold without prescriptions and the druggists had to recall the names of the customers. As an example, in East St. Louis, Illinois, forty-nine prescriptions were filled with limited identifications, such as first names only or names without addresses.

As a result of the relentless efforts of the FDA, 234 out of the 240 gallons produced were eventually retrieved, but by that time more than one hundred people, including many children, had died. Because the law of the time didn't prohibit the sale of toxic materials, Sam Massengill, the owner of the company, expressed his regrets but took no re-

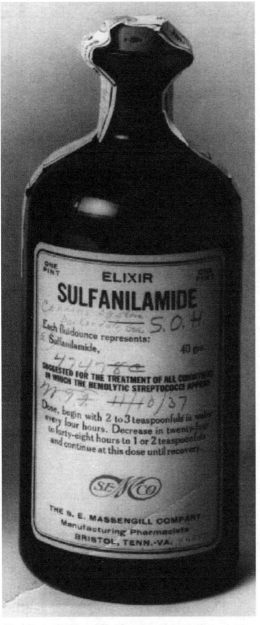

Bottle of Elixir Sulfanilamide taken from the FDA history Web site, http://www.fda.gov/cder/about/history/page18.htm (accessed July 28, 2005).

sponsibility for the manufacturing of the elixir, since he felt it was completely within the law. His chief chemist, however, did feel full accountability for this tragedy and committed suicide shortly after learning of the disastrous effects of his formulation.

The charge of illegally misbranding the product as an elixir was made simply because it contained no ethanol. Had the product been labeled "Solution Sulfanilamide" or "Liquid Sulfanilamide," no charges could have been made against the company.

The 1937 Elixir Sulfanilamide incident was widely reported in the press, and the outrage it generated directly led to the passage of the 1938 Food, Drug, and Cosmetic Act, which greatly expanded the FDA's authority to regulate the food and pharmaceutical industries and their products.

EVENT 13. TYPHOID MARY,
QUITE CONTRARY

Labels can be very powerful in evoking images. When a real estate development company buys up one hundred acres of "Dead Man's Gulch," and renames it "Harmony Mews," the land remains unchanged but our perception of it improves considerably. Coming across a reference to George Kelly or Lester Joseph Gillis would not kindle much interest for most readers. However, if they were referred to by their popular nicknames "Machine Gun" Kelly and "Baby Face Nelson," clearly identifiable images of violent prohibition gangsters would instantly appear in our mind's eye. Likewise, the name Mary Mallon means little to most people, but "Typhoid Mary" immediately conjures up the impression of a human carrier of death and disease.

However, a closer examination of the case of Mary Mallon reveals that the image we have is largely undeserved. Her story illustrates what can happen when the full weight of the establishment bears down upon a defenseless individual in order to set an example. The medical and scientific establishment singled out Mary Mallon as an archvillain in order to demonstrate their powers in service to the community—an act that was carried out with little sensitivity and no thought to the sanctity of individual rights and freedom. In truth, Typhoid Mary was far more a victim than a villain.

Typhoid fever is a life-threatening foodborne disease caused by bacteria of the Salmonella family—specifically *Salmonella typhi*. The spread of these bacteria is fairly straightforward and similar in many ways to other foodborne diseases. Infected people shed the typhoid bacteria in their urine and stools. The bacteria infiltrate the food and water system through direct contact with affected individuals or through untreated sewage wastewater. All you have to do is eat or drink contaminated products and reinfection is virtually guaranteed.

Typhoid bacteria enter the digestive tract, penetrate the lining of the intestines, and gain access to the bloodstream and underlying tissues. Inflammation of the small and large intestine follows. In severe infections, which can be life threatening, sores may develop in the small intestine. These sores bleed and sometimes perforate the intestinal wall. If the immune system is unable to stop the infection here, the bacteria will multiply and then spread to the bloodstream. *S. typhi* can be a very dangerous pathogen.

Symptoms usually begin to appear from eight to fourteen days after infection and include fever, headache, loss of appetite, sore throat, joint pain, constipation, and abdominal pain. As the disease progresses, fever often becomes very elevated and victims can become delirious. Fortunately modern antibiotic therapy can cure the disease, even though convalescence can take several months. At the turn of the last century, however, there was no cure, and the combination of rapidly growing cities and poor sanitation made typhoid fever one of the most dreaded of the urban diseases.

Starting in the 1880s, the United States saw an immigration explosion fueled by better economic prospects and the promise of freedom from political and religious persecution. With little more than the clothes on their backs, Italian, Irish, Polish, Eastern European, and Chinese immigrants entered the country in droves and inundated the poorest quarters of America's expanding cities. Not surprisingly, as the immigrant numbers rose, so did the racist attitudes of the country's established class. Immigrants were commonly stereotyped as being lazy, dirty, and untrustworthy.

Mary Mallon was born in County Tyrone, Ireland, in 1869, and immigrated to America about fifteen years later. Typical of the majority of immigrants at the time, she took on work as a domestic servant. While she may have started out doing menial labor such as washing and ironing, Mallon, by the beginning of the twentieth century, had risen to the rank of an established cook. This is a position that she must have been quite good at, because she was regularly employed in the homes of wealthy New York City families.

During the winter of 1906, George Soper, an 1899 graduate of Columbia's School of Mines program in sanitary engineering, was called in by George Thompson to investigate an outbreak of typhoid fever that had occurred several months earlier in a summer cottage he owned in Oyster Bay, Long Island. Thompson felt he would never be able to rent the cottage if the mystery of the outbreak could not be cleared up. In 1906 typhoid fever was not uncommon; 3,467 cases and 639 deaths were reported in New York City alone. However, Oyster Bay normally had very few, if any, cases.

Thompson had rented the house for the 1906 summer season to Charles Warren, a New York banker. On August 4, Warren hired Mary Mallon to replace the family's regular cook, whom he had discharged. Three weeks later, on August 27, Warren's daughter came down with typhoid fever, the first of several cases to appear in the household. In quick succession, two housemaids, Warren's wife, another daughter, and the gardener were all stricken with the disease. Fortunately, there were no fatalities.

Soper began by reviewing all of the studies that had been carried out during the original investigation by local health authorities, which immediately followed the outbreak. He found nothing to give any clear indication of the possible causes of the outbreak. He even followed up on the possibility that clams obtained locally might be the source of infection, but that trail led nowhere.

Since all the conventional sources of typhoid contamination, including water and milk, had been ruled out, he felt that some particular event preceding the first incident must have occurred in the household. He soon ascertained that the family's longtime cook had been replaced by Mary Mallon on August 4—a date that fit perfectly in with the outbreaks of the disease. In the paper he wrote for the *Journal of the American Medical Association* in 1907, Soper made his thoughts very clear: "Here was by all means the most important possibility in the way of a clue which had come to my notice. If this woman could be found and questioned, it seemed likely that she could give facts from which the cause of the epidemic could be ascertained."[11] He said almost the same thing in a paper he published in the *Military Surgeon Journal* twelve years later.

Thus, before ever meeting Mary Mallon, George Soper was fully convinced that he had found the individual associated with the origin of the typhoid fever outbreak. After he did track her down, he was extremely disappointed when she would not cooperate with him by providing samples of urine, feces, and blood. On the contrary, Mallon scared the wits out of Soper, to the point where he ran for his life: "It did not take Mary long to react to this suggestion. She seized a carving fork and advanced in my direction. I passed rapidly down the long narrow hall, through the tall iron gate, out through the area and so to the sidewalk. I felt rather lucky to escape."[12]

Since he could not get any information or samples from Mallon, he set about developing a history of her employment over the previous five years, confident that this would provide additional proof of her involvement in typhoid outbreaks. Even though he concluded that his study was only "partially satisfactory," he determined that seven out of the eight families he found had experienced outbreaks of typhoid fever during the period that Mary Mallon worked for them. Based on the results of this "shoe leather" epidemiological study, he immediately concluded that he had found the source of the outbreak.

In his article written thirty years later in the *Bulletin of the New York Academy of Medicine*, he said it best: "As a matter of fact, I did not need the specimens in order to prove that Mary was a focus of typhoid germs. My epidemiological evidence had proved that. Laboriously I had worked out every one of the seven outbreaks and I was positive that Mary had produced them all. Just exactly how she did it I didn't know."

With his study in hand, Soper went to the New York City health authorities and requested that Mallon be taken into custody and that samples of her feces, urine, and blood be collected and analyzed. This was immediately agreed to and, shortly thereafter, Dr. Josephine Baker was sent to get specimens of Mallon's blood and urine. Dr. Baker described Mallon as "a clean, neat, obviously self-respecting Irishwoman with a firm mouth and her hair done in a tight knot at the back of her head." Mallon refused to give any samples.

The next morning, accompanied by three policemen, Dr. Baker once more tried to get blood and urine samples, but the moment Mallon saw them she disappeared. It was several hours before they found her in a closet under the outside stairway leading to the front door of the house. She tried to put up a fight but was overwhelmed by the policeman who lifted her bodily into a waiting ambulance. Dr. Baker said that she was forced to sit on Mallon all the way to the hospital. Once Dr. Baker had Mallon in custody, she not only took blood and urine but samples of her bowel movements as well. It was in the latter samples that she found live cultures of typhoid bacteria. Later, Dr. Baker said: "And, to me, the interesting part of it all was that if Mary had let me have the specimens I was sent to get, she might have been a free woman all her life. It was her own bad behavior that inevitably led to her doom."[13]

Over the next two weeks, all but two samples of Mallon's feces revealed the presence of typhoid bacteria. Soper felt obliged to rationalize that the two samples that were negative were most likely too small. When reading Soper's papers, it is clear that he did not approach his study with cool detachment. He felt he had to pursue Mary Mallon much in the same way that Inspector Javert pursued Jean Valjean in *Les Misérables*. He staked his reputation on Mary Mallon as the person responsible for spreading typhoid fever.

Admittedly, Mary Mallon had much going against her. She was poor, she was an immigrant, she was Irish, and, possibly worst of all, she was a proud and independent woman. All of this in an age when most people in the establishment thought she should be obediently slaving away in a sweltering kitchen.

One can imagine Soper's shock when, earlier, after demanding samples of her feces, urine, and blood, she picked up a large fork and walked toward him. Here was a man who felt confident that he was the alpha male in this exchange, and all of a sudden Mallon had turned the tables on him. Such behavior did not fit the standards expected from a domestic servant—particularly a female one! He described his panicky flight as "passing rapidly down the long narrow hall." The whole affair might appear almost comical, but unfortunately, Mallon's pride and defiant independence ultimately worked against her.

Without a trial, a hearing, or legal representation of any kind, Mary Mallon was seized a few days later. In Soper's own words, "Mary Mallon was kept virtually a prisoner by the Department of Health for three years."[14] Soon after her capture, she was transferred to Riverside Hospital on North Brother Island in New York's East River—a hospital established to quarantine people with tuberculosis.

An innocent reference was made to "typhoid Mary" in a discussion of her case published in 1908 in the *Journal of the American Medical Association*.[15] Later in the same year, a textbook on typhoid fever used the same term, but this time it was capitalized as "Typhoid Mary."[16]

On June 20, 1909, one of William Randolph Hearst's sensationalist newspapers, the *New York American*, came out with a full two-page spread containing the banner headline "'Typhoid Mary' Most Harmless and Yet the Most Dangerous Woman in America." Smaller title lines on the page read "The Extraordinary Tale of Death and Disease Left by Mary Mallon" and "The Extraordinary Predicament of Mary Mallon, a Prisoner of New York's Quarantine Hospital Island, Not Because She Is Sick, but Because She Breeds Typhoid Fever Germs and Scatters Them Wherever She Goes."

The two-page spread was enhanced with photos of Mallon on North Brother Island and a profile sketch of people representing Mallon's victims. Rather than considering her case as a blatant miscarriage of justice, the paper sensationalized the dangers poor "Typhoid Mary" posed to the public at large. The most striking aspect of the article is a full page–length sketch showing Mallon cooking up eggs in a frying pan. Instead of eggs, however, five small skulls are seen being cooked! It was supposed to be a quasi-sympathetic article, but it could not have possibly done more damage to Mary Mallon. The mental construct any reader would make from that sketch was obvious—Mallon was a killer who used disease to carry out her dirty work.

Solely on the basis of her stool samples, Mallon was incarcerated and typecast as a chronic breeder of disease. None of the foods she prepared were ever tested nor were bacterial plate counts ever taken of her hands to demonstrate without question that she was not clean

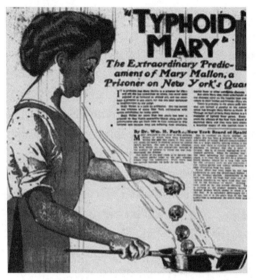

From "'Typhoid Mary,' Most Harmless and Yet the Most Dangerous Woman in America," *New York American*, June 20, 1909.

enough to work without spreading disease. There was nothing to explain the long periods of time when no disease occurred near her—an unusual circumstance for a chronic carrier.

In addition, it was known at the time that about 3 percent of individuals who contracted typhoid fever ended up being carriers. Estimates concluded that at the turn of the century somewhere from six thousand to nine thousand new asymptomatic carriers appeared each year in the United States. Only Typhoid Mary was imprisoned for suffering from that condition.

Two years after her initial detention, Mary Mallon sued the city of New York under a writ of habeas corpus for wrongful arrest. She was, after all, incarcerated without any due process and did not stand accused of committing any crime. Unfortunately, the judge dismissed the case by saying that the court was unwilling to take on the responsibility of releasing her. It was his version of Soper's "passing rapidly down the long narrow hall," and Mallon hadn't even approached him with a carving fork.

By the end of Mallon's third year of forced detention, the Health Department, under new supervision, released her on the condition that she agreed not to cook for her living. The affidavit she signed stated that she would agree to "take measures to protect any and all persons with whom I may come in contact from any infection," to which Mallon added the note "which it is possible I may cause." Despite the fact that her freedom relied entirely upon her signing the affidavit, Mallon stuck her neck out and insisted on adding her final word. Mary Mallon was still not convinced that she was responsible for all the outbreaks attributed to Typhoid Mary.

Soon after being released from captivity in 1910, Mallon disappeared and was not heard from for another five years. During this period, she worked in several places and, according to George Soper, produced "cases of typhoid . . . but there is no record of all of them."

During January and February of 1915, there was an outbreak of typhoid fever at the Sloan Hospital for Women in New York. The hospital's cook was a Mrs. Brown who had been nicknamed "Typhoid Mary" when the outbreak occurred. The hospital's head obstetrician, Dr. Cragin, called Soper and told him of the outbreak. Soper immediately dropped everything to go to the hospital. The cook wasn't there, so Dr. Cragin asked Soper to examine a note written by the cook. Soper immediately recognized the writing as that of Mary Mallon.

Mallon was quickly taken into custody and sent back to North Brother Island. There does not seem to be any record of a thorough investigation of the Sloan Hospital outbreak. The cause was presumed to be food that was consumed mainly by the physicians and nurses, who made up virtually all of the cases. However, several of the patients also ate the same food and did not get sick. It was immediately assumed that Mary Mallon was responsible. Three stool samples were taken for examination, but they were negative. A short time later, another sample was taken that turned out positive.[17] As a result, Mary Mallon was exiled for the remainder of her life because she violated the terms of her agreement—an agreement she objected to through the handwritten addition she made on the affidavit.

All in all, 47 cases of typhoid fever and 3 deaths were attributed to Mary Mallon. Another well-known carrier, Tony Labella, was responsible for 122 cases of typhoid fever and 5 deaths, but he was isolated for a total of two weeks and then released.

Mary Mallon remained on North Brother Island until her death in 1938. Five years before she passed away, she had a stroke that left her bedridden until death. She was buried by the New York Department of Health at Saint Raymond's Cemetery in the Bronx.

A month after Mallon died, George Soper wrote a typically self-serving letter to the *British Medical Journal* complaining of a flood of misstatements regarding "Typhoid Mary." He was particularly miffed at not receiving the appropriate credit for his "find": "The misstatements substitute a wholly imaginary account not only of the investigation itself but of the circumstances which led up to it, and rob me of whatever credit belongs to the discovery of the first typhoid carrier to be found in America and (to the time of her death) the most famous carrier anywhere."[18]

It remains unclear whether Mary Mallon was actually responsible for all the outbreaks attributed to her. The evidence against her was purely circumstantial, and the opportunities to develop a more definitive proof of her complicity were never taken. She very well may have been to blame, but this was not proven beyond a reasonable doubt.

In a statement far more sensitive and meaningful than George Soper's "Typhoid Mary" 1939 epitaph in the *British Medical Journal*, Dr. Josephine Baker, the person who first managed to take Mary Mallon into custody, soberly stated what Mallon was up against: "Typhoid Mary made me realize for the first time what sweeping powers are vested in Public Health authorities. There is very little that a Board of Health cannot do in the way of interfering with personal and property rights for the protection of the public health. Boards of Health have judicial, legislative and executive powers. . . . There have been many typhoid carriers recognized since her time but she was the first charted case and for that distinction she paid a life-long imprisonment."[19]

Mary Mallon was incarcerated for life without proof of her guilt beyond a reasonable doubt. There were an estimated six thousand to nine thousand other carriers of typhoid fever who were never incarcerated. Tony Labella, who was responsible for twice the number of incidents, was incarcerated for a total of two weeks. Given the foregoing travesty of justice, it's time for Typhoid Mary to be exonerated of the crimes she was accused of and for her name and reputation to be cleared.

EVENT 14. GINGER AILS

America has always been a hardworking and a hard-drinking country. By the 1830s, the annual per capita consumption of pure (100 percent) alcohol was estimated to be somewhere between five and ten gallons! The unfortunate social consequences of this kind of excessive drinking included increased physical abuse of spouses and children, violent crime, and poverty. Things got so bad that by the mid-1800s, several states formulated laws prohibiting or limiting the manufacture and sale of alcoholic beverages—except for medical purposes.

As a direct result of these laws and the growing temperance movement, alcohol consumption dropped considerably by 1860, but gradually began to creep back up after the Civil War. In reaction to this increase, thousands of women marched upon drinking establishments, singing and praying and creating enough havoc to make it pretty uncomfortable for the patrons and saloonkeepers—many of whom were forced to give up their businesses. By 1916 half of the states had adopted some form of antisaloon law, and in December of 1917, Congress submitted the Eighteenth Amendment to the Constitution, prohibiting "the manufacture, sale or transportation of intoxicating liquors." This was ratified in January 1919, with the approval of 80 percent of the forty-six state legislatures.

Nevertheless, the average per capita consumption was back up to almost seven gallons of alcohol each year—roughly equivalent to seventy quarts of whiskey for every person. Boozing it up was becoming a national epidemic. This called for drastic action, and to enforce the Eighteenth Amendment, Congressman Volstead of Minnesota introduced the National Prohibition Act, which Congress passed later in the year. Prohibition, the "Noble Experiment," was set in motion at the stroke of midnight on January 16, 1920, and from that moment on, it was illegal to manufacture beverages that contained more than 0.5 percent alcohol—except, of course, if it was for medicinal purposes.

Ah, the wonders of medicine! As far back as the mid-1800s, a well-known medicinal tonic was available in the United States that was simply an alcoholic extract of gingerroot. This preparation was supposedly used to aid digestion and to prevent respiratory infections. Because the extract was made from Jamaican ginger, it was nick-named "Jake" ginger. Oddly enough, in those parts of the country where local laws prohibited the sale of alcoholic beverages, people seemed to suffer most from digestive problems, because that's where Jake was most popular. Of course, another possible reason for Jake's popularity in those states was that it contained somewhere between 70 and 80 percent alcohol, making it a very strong, albeit disgusting, 150 proof beverage. The wonders of medicine, indeed!

Jake had always been considerably cheaper than normal whiskey because the alcohol used for its extraction was cheaper and taxed at a far lower rate. By itself, Jake was unpalatable because of the extremely high level of ginger extract (oleoresin) it was supposed to contain. This was not a major problem for most consumers, because they would simply dilute it with their favorite juice or soft drink.

After Prohibition came along, anyone who had money had very little trouble getting access to good-quality alcoholic beverages when-ever they wanted them. Poor people, however, couldn't afford these luxuries, and for those who needed alcohol, Jake was a cheap and con-venient alternative. In fact, Jake was a godsend for small-time boot-leggers during Prohibition. They did not have to compete with the vio-lent organized crime syndicates that dealt in decent booze and they had a large and steady market of paying customers, even if they didn't come from the upper layers of society.

Typically, Jake containing 70 percent alcohol was sold in two-ounce bottles for 50 cents and could be found for as low as three bottles for a dollar.[20] For any poor drinker, it was a real bargain, because you could make two pretty stiff drinks from one bottle. Jake could be found every-where in the South from pharmacies to grocery stores to gasoline stations—it could even be purchased in barbershops. It became so pop-ular during Prohibition that a song called "Jake Bottle Blues" was dedi-cated to it and recorded by Lemuel Turner in February 1928.[21]

In 1928 Harry Gross, a small-time bootlegger, rented the third and

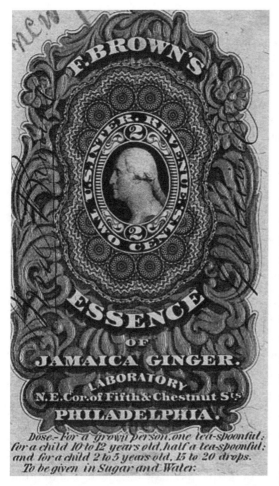

Label from an old bottle of Ginger Extract, photo by Morton Satin.

fourth floors of an old building at 65 Fulton Street in Boston from Louis Goldberg of the Central Wholesale Grocery Company. Harry referred to himself as a manufacturer and distributor of the medicinal product Fluid Extract of Ginger, and operated under the company name of the Hub Products Company. Although the manufacture of Jake was permitted, there were strict standards stipulating the minimum level of ginger oleoresin that had to be in the final product. The resulting fluid had such a strong taste and pungent aroma that it was almost undrinkable by itself, thereby limiting the amount that could be easily consumed. This was done on purpose because Jake was supposed to be a medicine, not an illegal replacement for whiskey.

However, when the government chemists checked products out, they never really analyzed for ginger as such. When they tested Jake, they simply heated it at 250°F for three hours in order to evaporate off all the alcohol and then weighed the oil and solids that remained. This residue was always presumed to be the ginger oleoresin, and if there was the proper amount left after the evaporation, the product passed the test. Since the primary focus of all the bootleggers was to produce the cheapest alcoholic product that could get around the Prohibition laws, this was an obvious invitation for bootleggers to adulterate Jake with anything that would not evaporate at 250°F. By doing this, they solved two problems: they could use much less of the expensive imported ginger extract and by reducing the ginger, they could make the product more palatable so people would drink more of it.

As a result, several bootleggers including Harry Gross began to adulterate Jake with other materials such as molasses and castor oil. In fact, in some cases the level of castor oil was so high that Jake ended up having a strong laxative effect. In retrospect, it is likely that this particular version of Jake was a very good cough remedy, because after you consumed it, you would be afraid to cough!

Ethanol, or drinking alcohol, has always had many industrial applications including perfumes, aftershaves, and a variety of other products. In order to control ethanol for the purposes of taxation, the government permits some of it to be "denatured," or purposely adulterated with small amounts of toxic chemicals such as methanol or acetone. This way, it couldn't be consumed as a beverage but was suitable for industrial purposes. During Prohibition, denatured alcohol was sold simply as an industrial solvent without the high taxes normally levied on drinking alcohol. This fostered a considerable illegal business designed to remove or "strip" the toxic chemicals out in order to resell the remaining ethanol to bootleggers as drinking alcohol. The problem was that it was extremely difficult to remove all the toxins, although that didn't seem to bother anybody in the bootlegging business. Thus stripped alcohol was commonly used by patent medicine manufacturers and bootleggers. Harry Gross may have bought his supplies from the Deluxe Drug Company in Brooklyn, New York, a company well known for the practice of alcohol stripping and one that also acted as a distributor of Hub Products' Jake.[22]

Using dubious-quality alcohol, bootleggers would add a bit of genuine ginger extract, castor oil, and molasses and end up with a cut-rate imitation of Jake that had some ginger flavor, but not enough to limit the amount that could be consumed. Best of all, if it was analyzed by government agents, it would test out just like genuine Jake.

The Jake business was always highly competitive, and since most consumers were not too particular about what they drank, the cheaper it could be made, the more competitive the product would be. By the end of 1929, the price of castor oil began to go up, and Harry Gross wanted to get a jump on his competitors. He had to find an alternative to replace castor oil if he was going to outdo the competition.

Working with Benjamin A. Werby, a chemist who was regularly consulted by bootleggers, Gross began searching for a castor oil replacement that could mix well with both the ginger oleoresin extract and the cheap alcohol he was using. During August and September of 1929, Hub Products purchased fifty-eight gallons of dibutyl phthalate, an oily liquid with a boiling point of 340°F. Dibutyl phthalate was normally used as an insect repellent, but Gross did not use it for long because of its obvious smell. He went back to castor oil, occasionally trying other materials such as butyl-carbitol or fusel oil, two rather obnoxious chemicals that evaporated too quickly to be of any practical use to him.

In early January 1930, Hub Products purchased a quantity of ethylene glycol from the company of Raffi and Swanson of Chelsea, Massachusetts. Ethylene glycol is the common antifreeze used in cooling and heating systems such as car radiators and constitutes a hazard when it is ingested. However, Gross found that much of it evaporated too quickly when put to the standard Jake test. He called Martin Swanson back and asked if he had anything similar that would not evaporate as quickly. Swanson would later maintain that he was a little perplexed because he couldn't understand how ethylene glycol could evaporate if it was used the way it was intended. Of course, Harry never admitted to Swanson what he was using it for.

Swanson then recommended another similar product called diethylene glycol, which was also used as an antifreeze. This had a higher evaporation point than ethylene glycol, but Gross decided to reject it because he felt that it also evaporated too quickly. He was looking for something that would not boil off at all during the evaporation test in case his Jake was checked out by government chemists. As it turned out, it was a good thing he rejected the diethylene glycol, because it is very toxic. In fact, eight years later, in a totally unrelated case, diethylene glycol was implicated in a highly publicized mass-poisoning outbreak that resulted in more than one hundred tragic deaths when it was used in a well-known medical elixir.[23]

Faced with a second rejection of material, Martin Swanson suggested to Gross that the only other thing he could recommend that would be less volatile than the diethylene glycol was a product called Lindol, the trade name for tri-ortho-cresyl phosphate (TCOP). Lindol was an oily, flame-resistant liquid that boiled at about 265°F—a perfect temperature to pass the standard Jake test. As it happened, Lindol was used in the preparation of lacquers and as a nonflammable fluid in hydraulic systems. Gross was very interested, and Martin Swanson personally brought the samples over to him.

A day later, on January 22, 1930, Swanson received a call from Benjamin Werby, Gross's chemist, asking about the toxicity of Lindol. Swanson had no information on this but said he would contact the Celluloid Company of Newark, New Jersey, the manufacturer of the product, to get the information. On January 24, Harry Gross ordered his first lot of Lindol from Raffi and Swanson—five gallons. Not having received a reply after three days, Werby called Swanson again, demanding that he immediately get the information on the toxicity of Lindol. The following day, Swanson called back, saying that the Celluloid Company believed the Lindol to be nontoxic. Gross immediately began ordering more Lindol from Raffi and Swanson—and ended up buying 135 gallons of it.[24]

It is interesting that Martin Swanson always maintained that he was totally unaware of the final intended use of the materials his company was supplying to Hub Products—a strange comment in light of the fact that he was also supplying them with ginger extract and that he had often visited the premises of Hub Products—where the only product made was Jake. In fact, when the Celluloid Company asked Swanson why he was inquiring about the toxicity of Lindol, Swanson fabricated the story that one of his employees swallowed some and he simply wanted to know if it was dangerous.

Harry Gross ran Hub Products like a very tight ship. Besides Harry, there were only two employees, a bookkeeper-stenographer named Miss Shirley Shapiro and Mr. George White, a young man who filled all the barrels and bottles with Jake and then shipped them out. Even though Hub Products occupied the third and fourth floors of 65 Fulton Street, these two employees were allowed only on the third floor. The fourth floor was the private domain of Harry Gross. Not even Benjamin Werby, his chemist, was allowed on that floor. In fact, Harry blocked all the entrances coming down from the fifth floor and going up from the third. He even made sure that no one could get in from the freight elevator. This was because the fourth floor was where Harry mixed his noxious brews—in complete secrecy—so that no one would ever learn his formulas or see what he was actually doing. When he finished concocting his adulterated Jake, Harry fed the blend into a rubber hose that snaked its way through a hole down to the third floor, where George White would fill the barrels or pack the product up into large, wholesale bottles, or the smaller, two-ounce retail ones. It was a crude but efficient setup, where only Harry really knew what was going on.

White first came to the attention of authorities when they noticed his signature on a delivery ticket for a barrel of Lindol originating from Raffi and Swanson. White told them that he would accept the Lindol from the Raffi and Swanson truck and then take it up to the third floor and leave it there. He went on to say that Gross would then take the Lindol to the fourth floor on the elevator by himself. White had no idea what Gross did with the Lindol, but he clearly stated that the empty barrels came down to the third floor again and were subsequently returned to Raffi and Swanson—indicating that Gross had used the product on the fourth floor. White went on to say that he would often see finished products on the third floor around quitting time, but when he returned the next day, they would be gone. He therefore presumed that Gross himself shipped a considerable amount of product out at night.[25]

Harry used several different company names to ship his products out, including the Standard Preserving Company, the Dominion Sales Company, Fulton Specialty Company, the International Sales Company, Phoenix Drug Company, and the Hub Products Company. In fact, he also got into an arrangement with a Mr. Austin E. Dolan to ship products under the name of the Dolan Drug and Chemical Company and the Dolan Drug Company in exchange for a payment of approximately fifty dollars per month.[26] Jake was distributed to customers all the way from New York to California, but mainly to distributors in Oklahoma, Tennessee, Missouri, Ohio, Kansas, and Kentucky.

With incredible rapidity, disturbing newspaper reports began to appear describing multiple cases of a strange new paralytic disease. On March 7, 1930, the *Daily Oklahoman* broke the story, but within two weeks, similar stories were appearing all over the country. Two physicians from Oklahoma, E. Miles and W. H. Goldfain, had already linked the paralysis to the ingestion of Jake Ginger, and all future stories confirmed this.[27] Within two weeks of drinking the Jake, victims would lose the feeling in their legs, experience weakness, and eventually suffer paralysis and "foot drop"—a condition where the foot hangs down limply when the leg is lifted. If this was not bad enough, victims continued to deteriorate through an almost identical set of symptoms occurring in the arms, complete with "wrist drop." Although few people died from consuming the bad Jake, recovery was extremely slow, and the majority of victims experienced some form of significant paralysis for the remainder of their lives.

Newspapers began to headline Jake Ginger paralysis stories. Here are some examples of articles just from the Boston area: "Two Men Paralyzed by Jamaica Ginger," "Poison in Ginger Drinks Discovered," "Wants Poison Ginger Seized," "Carbolic Acid Found in Drink," and "Poison Liquor Paralysis Gains."[28] An article titled "Police Seek Poisoned Liquor Source as 11 Paralysis Victims are Found" stated that

John J. MacNamara, age fifty, who had been arrested on charges of drunkenness, was gradually getting paralyzed while sitting in jail. When questioned, he said that his wife, Anna, had taken a drink from the same bottle. A visit to the home that day revealed that she, too, was becoming paralyzed.[29]

In mid-April, the paralysis began to reach epidemic proportions. No exact figures are available, but it has been estimated that more than fifty thousand Americans were left paralyzed by the bad Jake! In fact, the United Victims of Ginger Paralysis Association was eventually formed in order to try to get some form of compensation for their paralysis. The UVGPA had thirty-five members, leading to the opinion that as many as one hundred thousand people may have been poisoned before the materials were seized, since most people don't go through the trouble of joining such associations.

By May 1930, a whole collection of Jake songs began to emerge, all alluding to the epidemic of paralysis: "Jake Walk Blues," "Jake Leg Wobble," "Jake Leg Blues," and "Jake Leg Rag."[30] Jake drinkers were characterized as poverty-stricken, desperate trash. As a consequence, victims not only suffered from the paralysis itself but were also humiliated by the notoriety of this dreadful incident.

Drs. Maurice Smith and Elias Elvove of the National Institute of Health promptly confirmed the toxicity of the bad Jake, and the products were quickly traced back to the Hub Products Company at 65 Fulton Street in Boston. On March 17, 1930, FDA inspectors descended upon Hub Products, but Harry Gross was not particularly cooperative. He refused to talk to them without a lawyer. However, Harry was scared. His lawyer turned up later in the day at the FDA station in Boston and guaranteed that all shipments of the so-called Ginger Extract would be stopped immediately. As it turns out, as early as February 27, 1930, only three weeks after he started production of the Lindol-laced Jake, Gross must have known there was something horribly wrong with his product. He sent several drums of it to Atlas Storage under the name of Dolan Drug Company. Two days later, he instructed Atlas to get rid of the stuff, stating that "it was poison." It may be that he got word from one of the distributors that his Jake was paralyzing people.

Having ceased the production and shipment of Jake as of March 18, Gross moved lock, stock, and barrel out of 65 Fulton Street by April 10, 1930. Harry Gross, his brother-in-law Max Reisman (who financed part of Gross's operation), and Austin Dolan were quickly indicted in the federal courts of Kentucky, Ohio, and Kansas on the charge of conspiracy to violate the National Prohibition Act. Shortly thereafter, indictments were brought in to the Massachusetts Federal Court, on the charge of conspiracy to violate the National Prohibition Act as well as the Food and Drugs Act.

The defendants appeared before the court on March 2, 1931, a year after the mass poisonings had taken place. The defendants pleaded not guilty, but the trial was delayed due to the absence of the chosen judge. On April 10, Harry Gross changed his plea from not guilty to guilty, even though his attorneys argued that Harry was only a middleman. The judge bought his story, imposed a fine of one thousand dollars, and sentenced Gross to a two-year suspended sentence, putting him on probation with the proviso that he help the authorities trace and destroy all shipments and also find the "real" culprits, supposedly from New York. On May 4, 1931, Max Reisman also changed his plea to guilty and received a suspended two-year sentence, a condition of parole being that he, too, would help the authorities in their work. There does not appear to be any record on the outcome of the Dolan indictment, so presumably he was let off scot-free.

Even though the epidemic of Jake paralysis subsided by the fall of 1930, there was another large outbreak in California in January 1931. Apparently, some of Harry's products had been stored in Brooklyn. Local bootleggers added castor oil and sent it out to California.

Harry Gross and Max Reisman did nothing to assist in preventing the California outbreak, and Gross's story about the big boys of New York began to unravel in light of the ongoing investigation. This inspired the presiding judge to reconsider his original suspended sentence. Gross and Reisman were deemed to be in violation of their parole, and on April 1, 1932, Judge Lowell revoked the probation and sent the men to jail to serve out their sentences.

When Mr. H. M. Spillers, secretary of the United Victims of Ginger Paralysis Association, wrote to inquire as to the assets of Gross and Reisman, presumably to seek financial relief for his members, he was informed that they no longer had any property or bank accounts. They had never even paid their lawyers' fees.[31]

Not surprisingly, the FDA had always felt that both Raffi and Swanson, the suppliers of Lindol, and the chemist Benjamin Werby, may have been accessories to the conspiracy, but decided not to pursue the matter.

On Sunday, December 6, 1933, the *New York Times* ran the following story:

> Washington, Dec. 5 —Legal liquor today was returned to the United States, with President Roosevelt calling on the people to see that, "this return of individual freedom shall not be accompanied by the repugnant conditions that obtained prior to the adoption of the Eighteenth Amendment and those that have existed since its adoption."
>
> The new amendment repealed the Eighteenth, and with the demise of the latter went the Volstead Act which for more than a decade held legal drinks in America to less than one-half of 1 percent of alcohol and the enforcement of which cost more than 150 lives and billions in money.

There was no mention of the Ginger Jake paralysis victims anywhere in the text. It was as if the episode had never happened.

Perhaps the most shocking conclusion of the horrible Jake Ginger tragedy was that the man responsible for causing the lifelong paralysis of more than fifty thousand people was indicted only for conspiracy to sell illicit alcohol during Prohibition and for producing Jamaican Ginger Extract that did not comply with government regulations— nothing else. The massive poisoning he was responsible for was never addressed. Thousands upon thousands of people were left permanently crippled, impoverished, humiliated, and totally uncompensated, yet no individual seemed capable of gauging the full burden and significance of this reprehensible crime—except one.

A number of years after the appalling event, the following article appeared in a United Press clipping of October 1, 1936: "Harry Lesser, salesman of the 'ginger jake' that paralyzed many persons in Kansas City, Mo., and Boston during prohibition days, committed suicide by inhaling gas on August 31 in his home on Coney Island, it was learned today."[32]

Perhaps the most touching epitaph to the whole story was penned by the Allen Brothers in their song "The Jake Walk Blues":

> I can't eat,
> I can't talk
> Been drinking mean Jake, Lord
> Now I can't walk[33]

EVENT 15. MERCURY, THE MESSENGER OF FRAUDS

One of the most touching images I have ever seen appeared as the Picture of the Week in the June 2, 1972, edition of *Life* magazine.[34] The black-and-white image by renowned photographer Eugene W. Smith portrays a mother holding up her daughter in a traditional Japanese chamber bath. The look of anguish on the mother's face, the tender care with which she supports her daughter, and the heartbreaking pathos of the entire scene appears in my mind as a mirror image of Michelangelo's *Pietà* in St. Peter's Basilica.[35]

The caption on the photograph reads: "This is Tomoko Uemura. She was maimed by mercury poisoning in her mother's womb. Blind, speechless, crippled and deformed since birth, she must be bathed, fed and cared for like an infant. She is now 17."

One of the saddest aspects of this incredible photograph is the look on the face of Tomoko's mother. It almost appears as if she is saying to her daughter, "I'm sorry for what I've done to you."

The story of Tomoko Uemura is one of shame and disgrace. It involves the unconscionable behavior of a giant Japanese chemical corporation, the complicity of an uncaring government, and an indifferent public that simply preferred to look the other way.

The story unfolded in the tiny fishing village of Minamata on the western coast of southern Kyushu Island. The village was situated by a small bay of the same name in the Yatsushiro Sea. Minamata Bay was blessed with a natural reef that served as the spawning grounds for several species of fish and shellfish. As a result, the traditional village economy was based on fishing. Soon after the turn of the twentieth century, the company Nippon Chisso (Japan Nitrogen) built a chemical factory to produce fertilizer in the village.

In the 1930s, Chisso perfected a process to make acetaldehyde and various downstream products such as acetic acid, cellulose acetate, vinyl acetylene, and isooctane. In this process, acetylene is passed over a catalyst of mercury sulfate to produce acetaldehyde, which is then used to produce all the other derivatives. As the markets for these products grew, so did Chisso. As Chisso expanded, Minamata evolved from a quiet fishing village to a bustling town and finally to a small industrial city.

Unfortunately, Chisso's process of producing acetaldehyde resulted in a small portion of the mercury sulfate interacting with the acetylene to form organic compounds such as methylmercury. Since these organic mercury compounds had no value to Chisso, they were dumped together with all other waste products into the once pristine Minamata Bay. Because its commercial process was so profitable, Chisso quickly implemented it in its new operations in Korea and China. The town of Minamata continued to expand, even though the company policy of hiring the best people at the lowest possible wages never made anyone but Chisso's executives prosperous.

During the Second World War, Chisso made a fortune as a major supplier of strategic chemicals to the government. Unfortunately, Minamata Bay's stocks of fish and shellfish dwindled dramatically, making life very difficult for the local fishermen. Although it was never discussed openly, it was clear to nearly everyone that Chisso's practice of dumping its wastes into Minamata Bay was responsible for the loss of the fish and shellfish. The local fishermen's association went, cap in hand, to Chisso, asking for some type of compensation. The company gave them a pitiful one-time payment on the condition that no other demand would ever be made of them.

At the close of the war, Chisso lost all its offshore assets, as did many other giant Japanese corporations. However, the company made an incredibly rapid comeback because it produced ammonium sulfate fertilizer. Chisso, moreover, was in an ideal position to take advantage of the massive agricultural efforts to produce food in postwar Japan. Within two months of the war's end, Chisso was up and running at full steam. Although the company started out with ammonium sulfate production, it was not long before it was again producing acetaldehyde from acetylene. Shortly thereafter, Chisso began to produce polyvinyl chloride and dioctal phthalate (DOP—a general-purpose plasticizer) to supply the burgeoning international plastics market.

As Chisso's business grew, so did its toxic effluents, which it continued to dump into Minamata Bay without any treatment. By the mid-1950s, schools of dead or dying fish could be seen floating on the bay's surface. The reduced harvest impoverished the fishermen, forcing them to eat more of the products they caught. Once more, in desperation, they went to Chisso, asking for compensation. The company, trying to appear good-hearted and sympathetic, offered another pittance as long as the fishermen promised to cease all further claims against Chisso.

It was around this time that Minamata's inhabitants noticed a strange phenomenon. Local cats began to exhibit frenzied behavior, dancing and jumping awkwardly toward the bay. When they reached the water, they threw themselves in and drowned. They were appropriately called the "dancing suicide cats," but no one laughed at them. On the contrary, the bizarre behavior of the cats made people wonder if this was a premonition of bad things to come.

In May 1956, Minamata City Hospital (owned by the Chisso Corporation) admitted four patients who exhibited convulsions, agitated mental states, lapses into unconsciousness, coma, and finally death.

The hospital's director, Dr. Hosokawa, did a quick survey of the other medical facilities in the vicinity of the bay and found seventeen more fatalities with the same symptoms. The understanding in the local medical community was that this was not a new disease but one that had been going on for some time. Hosokawa started to make a record of it and asked staff at Kumamoto University in Kyushu to investigate. They quickly came to the conclusion that the fish and shellfish in Minamata Bay were poisonous.

Once more no one openly admitted it, but the answer was obvious to almost everyone—Chisso was poisoning the bay with its industrial wastes. How could anyone say anything against a giant of the chemical industry that was the city's economic base? No one did. Kumamoto's medical research group eventually determined that organic mercury in the waste stream was the primary cause of the disease, but Chisso quickly denied everything and severely criticized the quality of the university's research.

New cases of the disease were found in the nearby Fushimi Sea, where Chisso had redirected some of its waste effluent streams. There, too, a great many fish had died and the remainder was unsalable. Again the fishermen were forced to eat the fish they caught. By 1959 Chisso had effectively destroyed the fishing economy wherever its waste discharge pipes were located. Still, the company arrogantly denied any culpability, even though it provided the fishermen's associations of Minamata and Fushimi with token "sympathy" offerings.

Some fishermen were so incensed, they broke into Chisso's facilities and destroyed a few pieces of office equipment. This sort of behavior was unprecedented in Japan, and Chisso immediately brought in the police. The event was televised nationally, and the tragedy was finally brought to the country's attention—four years after the initial cases were admitted to Minamata Hospital.

Surprisingly, the fishermen received little sympathy from the public and even less from the government. After all, they had the audacity to criticize and attack an industrial giant that played a critical role in Japan's new economy. Such behavior was unheard of, and everyone immediately went into a form of denial, speculating on all sorts of other causes that might be responsible for Minamata disease.

Dr. Hosokawa continued to carry out a number of animal experiments and soon proved beyond doubt that Chisso's effluent was the singular cause of Minamata disease. The problem with Hosokawa's conclusions, however, was that he was not only director of the Minamata City Hospital, he was also the Chisso company doctor. When he presented his conclusive results to the company executives, they instructed him to immediately stop all research and ordered him not to disclose information to anyone. Since he was a loyal employee in the old tradition, Dr. Hosokawa politely bowed his head and sealed his lips until his deathbed.

By October 1959, Chisso was fully aware of its responsibility for the sickness and death of so many of the area's inhabitants and for the collapse of the local fisheries. Unfortunately, this knowledge didn't stop the company from continuing to dump toxic wastes into the local waters as it always had.

Mercury's toxicity depends on its form and route of exposure. When you swallow small amounts of liquid metal mercury, from a broken thermometer, for example, almost none of it will enter your body. Even if a person took in as much as a half pound (a little less than a tablespoon) of liquid mercury, very little absorption takes place. (I once heard a story that courtiers in Renaissance Europe used to swallow mercury and then have themselves turned over a number of times until it made its way through the gastrointestinal tract. Liquid mercury is so heavy you can apparently feel it moving through all the twists and turns of the intestine. It was supposed to be a form of courtly entertainment, but I haven't been able to verify this story anywhere in the literature.) Mercury vapors, on the other hand, are very toxic. When you breathe them in, about 80 percent of the mercury enters your bloodstream directly from your lungs and is quickly transported to other parts of your body, including the brain and kidneys. Once it makes it into your body, mercury can stay there for months.

Inorganic mercury salts such as mercurous nitrate and mercuric chloride do not vaporize at room temperatures as liquid metal mercury will. When inorganic mercury compounds are swallowed, less than 10 percent is usually absorbed. Lewis Carroll's "mad hatter" from *Alice in Wonderland* humorously portrayed the negative impact of mercury in the process of making hats. In fact, hatters really did go mad and develop severe and uncontrollable muscular tremors and twitching limbs, a condition called "hatter's shakes." Felt hats were made of fur, and the first step to making them was to apply a solution of mercurous nitrate to roughen up the hair fibers and make them mat together. The fibers were then shaved off the skin and converted to felt, which was later immersed in a hot acid solution. This acid treatment broke down the mercurous nitrate to metal mercury. The final step required steaming and ironing the hat, two hot processes that quickly vaporized the metal mercury and poisoned the hatters who invariably worked in poorly ventilated workshops.

While metallic mercury (unless vaporized) and metallic mercury salts have fairly low toxicities, organic mercury compounds, such as methylmercury, are extremely dangerous. They are readily absorbed into the body and can easily cross the blood-brain and placental barriers. These two body mechanisms evolved to prevent toxins from entering our nervous systems and to protect a growing fetus. Unfortunately, methylmercury combines with one amino acid (cysteine) and tricks these defense mechanisms into thinking it is another amino acid (methionine). Once it crosses these defensive barriers, it is in the brain and central nervous system where methylmercury does its greatest damage—it destroys nerve cells, which results in devastating neurological problems.

In the fetus, methylmercury interferes with nerve cell development by binding to DNA. It also interferes with normal brain development. Exposure, while in the womb, can result in small misshapen heads, mental retardation, cerebral palsy, blindness, deafness, and seizures. As in the case of Tomoko Uemura, affected children can be born to mothers who exhibited no symptoms of methylmercury poisoning during their pregnancy.

Chisso knew all this, but chose to continue dumping its toxic wastes into Minamata Bay. The plankton and shellfish took it up, fish ate the plankton, bigger fish ate the smaller fish, and people ate the fish and shellfish.

Methylmercury bioaccumulates as it moves up the food chain so that the levels found in animals and people can be several million times higher than in the waters from which the consumed fish were taken. Like the rest of Japan, the diet of the people in Minamata depended largely on fish and shellfish for protein. The levels of mercury in their bodies climbed steadily because they had no other options but to eat the fish from the bay.

So many people were affected and so many babies were born disabled that by the end of 1959, the governor of the prefecture had no choice but to intervene and order Chisso to pay ¥100 million to the fishermen's associations. This might sound like a lot of money, but in 1959 it was the equivalent of only $28,000 in US dollars. The Minamata Disease Association paid $830 for each confirmed death and $280 for every survivor, regardless of how grievous the symptoms were.

Chisso insisted that these payments in no way reflected any responsibility on its part. The company claimed to be just good corporate citizens providing a gift of condolence to people who fell upon misfortune. It also added a clause prohibiting any further claims against the company. If anyone else became ill, the government would have to compensate them. All the while, Chisso's stream of toxic effluent continued to pour into the bay and surrounding waters.

Despite the fact that the government cut off funds for further mercury research, Kumamoto University continued to study the subject and, in 1962, demonstrated publicly for the first time that methylmercury was produced as a result of Chisso's acetaldehyde process—a fact that was long known by the company but kept secret. As soon as Kumamoto's results were made public, Chisso immediately objected and claimed that the university's research was bogus.

Chisso kept a lid on things until 1965, when a rash of new cases was reported in Niigata City, far from Minamata. It did not take long for Kumamoto University researchers to pinpoint the problem: toxic waste discharge from another acetaldehyde plant, this time owned by the Showa Denko Company. In lockstep with Chisso, Showa Denko denied all responsibility, but by this time the dancing cats were out of the bag.

A lawsuit was brought by the Miike family—poor fishermen whose extended family had suffered grievously from eating the poisoned fish and shellfish. In 1968, the Japanese government finally gave official recognition to the direct relationship between methylmercury in the toxic waste streams and Minamata disease—a dozen years after the cause was first uncovered.

After protracted negotiations, the victims received a more reasonable compensation package, but most of this was paid for by the government, not Chisso. The *Japan Times* recently reported on government plans to financially assist three thousand Minamata disease victims of the 1950s and 1960s. This decision was finally made in April 2005, fifty years after the first victims entered Minamata City Hospital!

On his deathbed, Dr. Hosokawa testified that all his research—proving the link between methylmercury and Minamata disease—was kept secret or destroyed by the Chisso Corporation. Tomoko Uemura died in 1977, five years after photographer Eugene Smith produced the stunning image that is considered to be one of the hundred most influential photos ever taken.

EVENT 16. THE DRAIN IN SPAIN

On May 1, 1981, an eight-year-old boy, Jaime Vaquero Garcia, died on the way to Madrid's La Paz Children's Hospital. Soon afterward, five of Jaime's brothers and sisters were examined at the same hospital and found to be very ill. Symptoms included interstitial pulmonary infiltrate (congested lungs), headache, weakness, scalp itchiness, and slight fever. They were initially diagnosed as having atypical pneumonia. The doctors immediately put one of the girls into intensive care, and the other four children were transferred to the Hospital del Rey, Madrid's well-known institution for infectious diseases.

Within days the number of patients admitted to hospitals all over Madrid began to rise meteorically.

Politically, it was an extremely sensitive period in Spain. The country had just begun to experience democracy after General Francisco Franco's forty years of fascist dictatorship ended in 1975. Three months before the outbreak began, a senior army officer made an unsuccessful attempt to restore military rule by holding members of parliament at gunpoint. Dealing with a major epidemic of illness across the country was the last thing anyone needed.

Because of the victims' symptoms, the hunt for some type of infectious agent immediately began. Early in the epidemic, the clinical picture supported the search for an infectious agent as the cause of the illness. Because of political and social pressures, the Spanish government immediately diverted scarce medical resources to investigate the cause based on the infectious hypothesis. The clinicians at a Madrid pediatric hospital compared children treated with erythromycin to groups who received other treatments, including antihistamines, other antibiotics, and placebos, but they found that the evolution of the epidemic's symptoms was similar in all groups.[36]

The acute phase of the disease was characterized by noncardiogenic pulmonary edema (changes to the pulmonary capillary membrane) with headaches, asthenia, itchy scalp, rash, abdominal pain, and fever. Severe muscle pain and cramps marked the end of the acute phase. After the first two months, patients entered an intermediate phase, which seemed to last another two months. The clinical features of this phase were characterized by abnormalities of the sensory nervous system and intense muscle pain. Other symptoms included difficulty in swallowing, pulmonary hypertension, deposition of blood clots in the large vessels, marked weight loss, increased levels of peripheral red blood cells, and elevated triglycerides and cholesterol.

Almost 60 percent of the patients went on to a chronic phase with pathological thickening and hardening of the skin, motor and sensory nerve degeneration, carpal tunnel syndrome, and muscle pain and cramps. Problems such as memory loss and depression were also reported during the chronic phase.[37]

Dr. Manuel Tabuenca, a pediatrician at the Hospital Infantil de Niño Jesus, soon informed the government that he had finally determined the cause of the epidemic. He had investigated 210 of the children under his care and found that all had consumed cooking oil. This study established that consumption of oil sold in unlabeled five-liter plastic containers was a clear risk factor for developing this epidemic syndrome.

Following this finding, oils collected from affected households and open-air markets were analyzed by the government laboratory. The oil in question turned out to be rapeseed oil rather than olive oil, which is what the affected people thought they had bought.

Although the edible form of rapeseed oil is currently accepted as excellent food oil, this was not always the case. Traditional rapeseed oil contains high levels of erucic acid, which has been linked to the formation of fatty deposits in heart muscle and the consequent negative cardiac events. It also contains high levels of glucosinolates, which are toxic antinutritional compounds. After extensive research, Canadian plant breeders were able to develop an oil that had extremely low levels of both these compounds—a product we now know as canola oil.

But it was the old version of rapeseed oil that was implicated in the Spanish outbreak. In fact, erucic acid had excellent lubricating properties, which made the traditional rapeseed oil ideal for industrial uses—but not very good for food use. This was why the potent toxin aniline was added as a denaturant—so people would not use the oil in food. But, like the alcohol strippers of the Prohibition, there were operators who made a living stripping the aniline out of rapeseed oil so that it could be used as a cheap food oil substitute.

The rapeseed oils found by the Madrid medical researchers were originally denatured with 2 percent aniline but now contained other aniline-derived compounds. This indicated that they had been reprocessed and reheated. (It was later learned that the Spanish customs laboratory had known of the importation of aniline-denatured rapeseed oil for several months.) On June 10, 1981, exactly forty days after the epidemic began, an official announcement was made by the Ministry of Health and Consumer Affairs on late-night television, informing the public that the widespread epidemic had been the result of contaminated, unlabeled cooking oil.

Referring to the outbreak as Toxic Oil Syndrome, or TOS, the announcement stated that the hospitals remained full of victims. But after the announcement, new admissions precipitously dropped. All suspected supplies of toxic oil would be recalled. Overnight, the panic that had gripped the country for weeks subsided.

The number of cases continued to drop after the oil recall was instituted. By October 1981, almost no cases were reported. By the time the outbreak was quelled, more than twenty thousand people were diagnosed with acute TOS. About 59 percent of those affected progressed to a chronic stage of the disease and had to be hospitalized with symptoms including neurological deficiencies, carpal tunnel syndrome, and muscle cramps. Approximately 375 deaths were reported, but that was only the beginning.

Through the combined efforts of the Centers for Disease Control and Prevention in Atlanta, the department of biological sciences and human oncology at the University of Turin, and the Servicio de Información Sanitaria in Madrid, a detailed follow-up by telephone or mail to almost every living member of the affected families revealed that from May 1981 through the end of December 1994, the actual number of deaths amounted to 1,663![38] The Spanish Toxic Oil Syndrome must therefore go down in history as one of the most lethal food-poisoning events.

A full eighteen years after exposure to the toxic oil, surviving victims continued to suffer from profound neurological disorders, including decreased sense of touch and muscle weakness. In addition, as was the case with the Ginger Jake affair, the affected victims were further stigmatized for being of the poor lower classes.

Nevertheless, the victims took the government to court, and indemnities were established by the Supreme Court in 1997 at a major cost amounting to more than three hundred million euros by 2002. Current regular payments to beneficiaries come to about twenty million euros per year.

Many oil merchants were arrested soon after it was concluded that oil was the responsible agent. By 1987 these merchants were brought to trial. The trial lasted two years and resulted in the conviction and imprisonment of a number of the accused, even though the judges stressed that the actual toxin in the oil that caused the disease was still not fully known. In fact, that remains the case today.

This has led some to believe that the published material was nothing but a massive cover-up by the government and scientific establishment. Bob Woffinden, an investigative reporter for the British newspaper the *Guardian*, has built a case on the premise that cooking oil had nothing to do with the outbreak, but that organophosphate pesticides were the responsible agents.[39]

Despite all the controversy, research continues into finding the most likely toxic compounds that might have caused the disaster, but there are no definitive answers as yet.

EVENT 17. IN VINO VERITOX

Years ago, while living in Italy, my wife and I decided to join one of the diplomatic community's cosmopolitan wine groups. Since my wine tastes were not quite in keeping with the rather refined tastes of this group, I decided to read whatever I could about wine and then make a conscious effort to carry on sophisticated wine babble at these get-togethers. It didn't take long before I was able to comfortably say things like, "This vintage appears to be a naive little Carmignano with very little breeding, but I'm rather amused by its fruitless presumption" or "I really find the nose of this wine needlessly arrogant and its backbone somewhat obtuse, but I'm rather taken with its voluptuous conjecture. Gauche, n'est pas?"

There are few things in life that bring out snobbery like wine does.

Yet, as was seen in the section on lead poisoning, wine has been the object of continual adulteration from the time it was first invented through today. Alcoholic beverages including wines are among the least transparent products available to consumers. We all read of the grapes being grown in small vineyards on the slope of a hill, where water slowly trickles down at the perfect angle to result in the optimal moisture to give the wine its magnificent body. But we never hear of the winemeister dumping flocculating agents, bentonite, erythorbic acid, hydrogen peroxide, isinglass, potassium ferrocyanide, polyvinyl-polypyrrolidone, or potassium metabisulphite into the vat—all of which are perfectly legal.

It is difficult to understand why alcoholic beverages have managed to escape the watchful eye of government regulators in terms of consumer labeling. Aside from the obvious reasons that the alcohol industry is an excellent source of tax revenue as well as supporting a very effective lobbying effort, it is likely that most consumers want to know as little of the nitty-gritty of alcoholic beverages as possible. Perhaps it is because we are content to retain a certain mystique when it comes to products such as wine, beer, and whiskey. The problem with keeping this sort of distance is that we are susceptible to manufacturers who might cut corners and make cheap, low-quality products appear to be higher in quality than they actually are.

Fake or adulterated wines or whiskeys constitute anywhere from 5 to 10 percent of the current worldwide market. The percentage is far greater in newly emerging economies where the burgeoning middle and upper classes wish to flaunt their wealth by emulating their Western counterparts. China and Thailand are excellent examples. In 2005 a Beijing supermarket proudly displayed a tall, thin bottle of "Whistler Estates" Canadian ice wine on its wine shelves. Not satisfied with simply using the name of Canada's top ski resort north of Vancouver, the bottler placed an additional label on the same bottle, referring to "Niagara Fall Pensula [sic]" and another smaller label, "Rocky Mountain ice wine." It was some time before the fake wine, complete with its misspelled labels, was discovered. In the interim, Chinese new wine connoisseurs with far more money than taste happily paid forty to eighty dollars a bottle (more than the average monthly wage of a Chinese worker) for a concoction that experts claimed tasted like bad cough medicine.

Wine has always had its fraudulent side. Geoffrey Chaucer warned in his fourteenth-century *Canterbury Tales*, "Keep clear of wine, I tell you, white or red, especially Spanish wines, which they provide and have on sale in Fish Street and Cheapside. That wine mysteriously finds its way to mix itself with others."

John Calvin wrote that there were so many parts of the true Christian cross that "whereas the original cross could be carried by one man, it would take three hundred men to support the weight of the existing fragments of it." In the same way, the volume of 1947 first-growth vintages sold in recent years exceeded the whole year's production. Producers of one of the world's most famous wines, Sassicaia, were forced to redesign their bottles after the fraudulent production and sale of twenty thousand bottles designed to look just like their product. A similar fraud occurred with Australia's famous Penfolds Grange wines. It is no surprise that the higher the price of the wine, the greater the profit for counterfeiters and the less likelihood that the victims would be willing to admit to their error.

Perhaps the most famous wine fraud in recent history was the Austrian antifreeze scandal of 1985. In fact, the scandal started a decade earlier when an enterprising biochemist decided to concoct a formula for artificial wine out of various chemicals. While the finished product did indeed resemble wine, he found that it was more expensive to make than wine using the natural winemaking process. A key ingredient in his formula, which added both sweetness and body to the final product, was diethylene glycol. Diethylene glycol is highly soluble in water and can be found in the radiators of most cars, trucks, and tractors, because it is a perfect antifreeze in hot and cold climates. Diethylene glycol is also highly toxic and is the very same material that caused the 107 deaths in the 1937 Elixir Sulfanilamide disaster in the United States.

When the scientist found that his chemical wine could not compete, he looked into the idea of upgrading cheap wines into sweeter varieties with more body so that they could compete with higher-priced varieties. Despite his being the cellar master of a large and well-known Austrian wine firm, he ignored the fact that diethylene glycol was a highly toxic material. He then proceeded to sell the secret to several other wine growers and dealers in Austria, who were then able to transform their cheap wines into expensive ones through this adulteration. As original as our modern-day chemist thought he was being, the Greeks and Romans had done almost the same thing two thousand years earlier with sapa. The difference was that the new diethylene glycol could be toxic!

Although the levels of diethylene glycol added were not high enough to poison anyone immediately, it was an adulteration of the worst type. This scandal went on for a number of years and would have continued were it not for the excessive greed and stupidity of one of the winemakers—and there is always one. Not satisfied that he was making exorbitant profits through his adulteration efforts, the individual tried to get a refund on the tax he had paid on a very large quantity of diethylene glycol. This alerted the local tax inspector, who could not imagine why this person needed the diethylene glycol. The inspector reported the suspicious act to ministry officials in Vienna in December 1984.

Within six months, the Austrian police arrested all the key suspects. They seized almost five million liters of contaminated wines, some going back to 1976. They were the sweet varieties familiar to anyone who drank Austrian wine: Spätlese, Auslese, Beerenauslese, Trockenbeerenauslese, and even an Eiswein. It proved to be a disaster for the Austrian wine industry. Even though a relatively small proportion of Austrian wines were involved, all wines were now considered suspect. Austrian wine exports collapsed. In an interesting twist, German wine importers wanted to return all wines and employed chemical tests to demonstrate that German wines were free of diethylene glycol. Unfortunately, several of their own wines failed the test, indicating that a number of bottlers had illegally mixed Austrian wines together with their native German products.

Although the Austrian wine adulteration was a great scandal and wreaked havoc upon the industry, there was not a single fatality reported as a result of drinking the doctored products. Although diethylene glycol is toxic, the levels added were low enough that an individual would have to have consumed twenty-four bottles to experience a toxic reaction.

Not to be outdone by the Austrian wine adulterers, a number of wine producers from the Piedmont region of northern Italy decided to run a wine-adulteration scam of their own. Braced by the Italian Alps to the north and the wooded Apennine Mountains to the south, Piedmont has long been known for its rich culture and the superb wines it produces from its two major wine-growing areas: Alba in the southwest and Asti in the southeast.

The Asti region is most famous for sparkling wines such as Asti Spumante or the distinctive, sweet, nonsparkling Moscatos. Here you can also find the excellent Barbera d'Asti, which is not as robust as its Barbera d'Alba cohort. In Alba, you find Italy's big B's: Barolo, Barbaresco, and Barbera. For a lighter wine, Alba also produces the delicious Dolcetto—a red wine that has the light body and fruity aroma of the best whites.

With all this natural bounty and a ready market for all wine products, you would think that winemakers would be delighted with the status quo—but that was not the case for everyone.

The Italian wine scandal broke on March 18, 1986. This scandal involved the adulteration of Piedmont wines with toxic materials that resulted in the deaths of twenty-five individuals and the hospitalization of many others. The investigation that followed found that in December 1985 approximately thirty of the region's wine producers blended their wines with toxic amounts of methanol, a compound often used in much smaller quantities to increase a poor wine's alcohol level. In these wines, however, the levels of toxic methanol were as high as 5.7 percent—almost twenty times higher than the permitted level of 0.3 percent! Most of the wine had been sold in bulk to the cheaper wine bars and groceterias where less wealthy people shopped to fill up their demijohns for home consumption.

Filippo Pandolfi, the Italian minister of agriculture, fearing catastrophic damage to Italy's wine industry, quickly announced new regulations requiring all export wines to carry an official certificate of purity. Italy's biggest wine-growing association guaranteed that no adulterated wine was ever exported to the United States, the country's largest export market. The European market was unable to get the same assurance because millions of gallons had already been shipped to France and Germany. Fortunately, the shipment was confiscated in time and no further mortalities occurred.

The Italian carabinieri arrested Giovanni Ciravegna and his son Daniele on multiple charges of manslaughter. The elder Ciravegna received fourteen years imprisonment for his efforts. Eleven other stiff sentences were meted out by the Italian courts. An association of victims was established to get compensation for all those affected—and there were many. Methanol has many toxic outcomes including permanent blindness and ataxia (loss of coordination). Unfortunately, the only thing these victims received from the government thus far has been promises.

The Italian wine industry fared much better than the victims. As a result of an increased effort to improve quality, sales of Italian wines have skyrocketed. Exports to the United States now exceed a billion dollars a year (even though it is estimated that the sales of counterfeit Italian wines is almost the same as that of genuine imports—in other words, one out of every two bottles of "Italian" wine may be a fake![40]

Methanol poisoning from adulterated alcoholic beverages continues all around the world. In September of 1999, Kenyan officials reported the deaths of twenty-three people in the Embu district as a result of consuming methanol in liquor disguised as whiskey. This was neither the first nor is it likely to be the last occurrence of this problem in Kenya. Eighty people died in August 1998 after drinking another illegal brew that was contaminated with methanol in the western Nakuru district. Again, in November 2000, more than 130 individuals died and more than 500 were hospitalized with permanent disabilities from drinking methanol-laced liquor. Not surprisingly, all the victims were from a poor Nairobi slum district.

In October 2000, a methanol poisoning epidemic left 117 people dead and many blind in El Salvador. Most victims were poor farm-workers from San Vicente, a small city sixty kilometers from San Salvador, the country's capital. They had all consumed the popular sugar-cane liquor called Trueno or Thunderbolt. The scammers simply refilled old Thunderbolt bottles with diluted industrial-grade methanol.

In Estonia in 2001, a group of swindlers found a drum of industrial-grade methyl alcohol. Taking advantage of their prize, they diluted it with water, bottled the mixture, and sold it as cheap vodka—not a good idea in a country where alcoholism is a chronic problem. Within a few days, sixty-seven people were dead and many others hospitalized.

More recently, in 2004, nine people died from drinking wine laced with methanol in Guangzhou, the capital of South China's Guangdong Province. Several others were hospitalized with the severe symptoms typical of methanol intoxication. Local police detained a dozen suspects and accused them of blending industrial methanol with rice wine before selling it to local markets.

No doubt there are dozens more cases of methanol poisoning around the world that go unreported. As long as the global wine and spirits industry is allowed to hide its ingredients and additives, it is an open invitation for abuse and adulteration. Without greater transparency, the opportunities for chronic intoxication and poisoning are greatly increased.

EVENT 18. FUGU FISH—BONZAI OR ZOMBIE?

> Those who eat fugu soup are stupid.
> But those who don't eat fugu soup are also stupid.
> Traditional Japanese expression[41]

Fugu is the Japanese name for the odd-looking puffer fish. Fugu are highly toxic fish, but the Japanese consider it to be a great delicacy for those who can afford to eat it. Lethal amounts of the poison tetrodotoxin are concentrated in the fish's liver, gonads, and skin. For a long time, the origin of the fugu's tetrodotoxin was a scientific mystery, with some scholars arguing that the poison was produced by the fish's body. However, it is now believed that the tetrodotoxin derives from bacteria associated with the fish and the marine organisms it eats.

Because fugu toxin is a thousand times more poisonous than cyanide, only specially licensed chefs are allowed to prepare it. Obtaining a license to prepare fugu is a ten-year process, involving several varieties of puffer fish. It is such a stressful and exhausting process that once they have completed the course, chefs are supposedly able to hear the final lament of the puffer fish laid out on the chopping block.

When I visited the Marine Biotechnology Institute in Kamaishi, Japan, a number of years ago, I was invited out for sashimi, of which I am very fond. During the middle of the meal, my host asked me if I was interested in trying some fugu. I jumped at the opportunity. When it came, I savored it slowly, but was rather disappointed in it. While I desperately looked for subtle nuances in flavor and texture, I found none. Of course, I did not say this to my host. I simply presumed that I did not have the experience or sophistication to appreciate its special qualities. Considering that an average serving of fugu can cost anything from thirty to two hundred dollars a plate, I decided that its

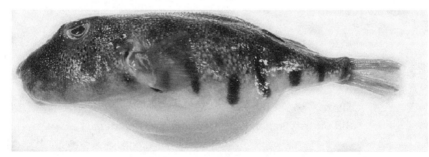

Puffer fish, photo taken in Tokyo's Tsukiji Market by Morton Satin.

appeal to the Japanese would remain a mystery to me.

Some time later, I mentioned this disappointing experience to a close Japanese colleague. He immediately started to laugh. "People don't eat it for the taste or texture," he said. "They eat it in order to flirt with death! Of course, they say it is delicious, but it is the poison they are after." I looked at him, a bit dumbfounded. "It starts with a tingling of the lips, and a bit of a buzz in the head—then if you have a really good chef, you will begin to feel tightness in the chest and have difficulty breathing. Your head will feel hot and you will have trouble keeping your eyes in focus. If your chef is great, and has served you before and knows how much you can handle, you might even pass out for a few hours! You see, it is not the job of the fugu chef to remove all of the toxin. It is his job to leave in just enough toxin to provide you with the excitement you desire."

Typically, the first symptoms of poisoning occur between fifteen minutes and several hours after eating fugu. Initial symptoms include the tingling of tongue and lips, quickly followed by facial numbness. Salivation, nausea, vomiting, and diarrhea with some abdominal pain develop early. Motor dysfunction with muscle weakness, hypoventilation, and speech difficulties then develop. A rapid ascending paralysis occurs over four to twenty-four hours. Extremity paralysis is followed by respiratory muscle paralysis. Finally, the victim experiences cardiac dysfunction along with central nervous system dysfunction (e.g., coma), and seizures can develop. Patients with severe toxicity may have a deep coma, fixed nonreactive pupils, apnea, and loss of all brain stem reflexes. In other cases, one might experience all the paralytic physical functions yet still be able to see and think very clearly. Death can occur within four to six hours as a result of respiratory muscle paralysis and respiratory failure.

The only advantage of an early onset of symptoms is that the diner can get out of paying the outrageous cost of the dish!

Every year, because of miscalculations in the amount of poison left in the fugu fish, several hundred people are poisoned (with twenty to one hundred fatalities) in Japan.[42] According to records, 1958 was a banner year, with 176 fugu deaths occurring throughout Japan. The most famous victim was the Kabuki actor Bando Mitsugoro VIII, who had achieved the status of a Living National Treasure. He expired in a Kyoto restaurant in 1975 after gorging himself on four bowls of *chiri*, a broth containing pieces of poisonous fugu liver. Considering that fugu consumption in Japan has been traced back to the Jomon period (ca. 10,000–300 BCE), Mitsugora Bando's death followed a long tradition.

Fugu consumption was largely banned in Japan from the sixteenth to the nineteenth century because of all the lives it claimed. However, Japan's first prime minister, Hirobumi Ito (1841–1909), the man responsible for the modernization of Japan, was also responsible for putting fugu back on the traditional Japanese menu. When he first tried it, Ito was so taken with its taste that he ordered the resumption of fugu preparation and sale.

While it is one thing to voluntarily consume tetrodotoxin for the thrill of flirting with death, it is entirely another matter to deliberately poison someone. In one of the more bizarre toxicological discoveries of the twentieth century, fugu fish has been implicated with the Haitian practice of voodoo and the supposed existence of zombies.

The affair began in Haiti in 1962 when Clairvius Narcisse disagreed with his brothers and refused to sell his share of the family land. In order to get rid of him, his brothers sold Clairvius to a witch doctor, who apparently fed him a concoction designed to turn him into a zombie. On April 30, 1962, Narcisse stumbled into the emergency room of the American-run Schweitzer Hospital. He was feverish and spitting up blood. He appeared to be suffering from malnutrition and fever and complained of aches throughout his body. The doctors were unable to diagnose his illness, and his condition deteriorated rapidly. He developed respiratory problems and then slipped into a coma.[43] According to hospital records, he died three days after he entered the hospital. Attending physicians (including one American) signed his formal death certificate. No autopsy was made, and his body was placed in cold storage for twenty hours before his burial.

Narcisse next turned up in 1980, when he accidentally stumbled across his long-lost sister in a marketplace. Not surprisingly, she didn't recognize him, but then he told her his boyhood nickname and personal facts that only intimate family members would know. She couldn't believe it—she had attended his funeral eighteen years earlier! Clairvius said he remembered the color of the dress she wore to his funeral. Other villagers soon recognized him.

He told her that when he was lowered into his grave, he was fully conscious, but unable to move or utter any sound. When earth was thrown over his coffin, he envisioned everything as if he were floating above it all. He pointed to the scar on his right cheek and told her it was from a nail carelessly driven through the casket.

During the night, a voodoo priest came and, after digging out his coffin, raised him from the dead. He was beaten, tied up, and taken to a sugar plantation in northern Haiti where, along with others who suffered a similar fate, he was made to work as a slave—a zombie slave. In 1964 the zombie master died and the slaves escaped the plantation and dispersed throughout the island in a psychotic daze. It was only by accident that Narcisse stumbled across his sister in the market. No one doubted his story because there is a strong belief in voodoo and its effects throughout Haiti.

The story was written up in a number of well-known magazines and attracted the attention of a group of people interested in determining its authenticity and the material responsible for causing someone to become one of the living dead. A young Canadian ethnobotany graduate student at Harvard, Wade Davis, was dispatched to Haiti to "get the goods" on zombies.

After some time, Davis was able to acquire a number of samples of powders that were supposed to be able to turn people into zombies. Upon analysis, it was found that they all contained tetrodotoxin—the very same poison in the fugu for which Japanese diners pay two hundred dollars a plate. When tetrodotoxin was given to laboratory rats, they became comatose and appeared to be dead, but their EKGs showed a faint heartbeat and the EEGs detected the presence of brain waves. Although it was theorized that this was a clear demonstration of the ability of "zombie powder" to induce a comatose state, the experiment could never be repeated. In fact, the individual who carried out the original research declined comment on the results and refused to have any further contact with Davis—never a particularly good sign when trying to confirm a story.

In the cold light of scientific scrutiny, the evidence supporting the zombie powder theory is pretty weak. That is not to say that it is totally out of the question. In a highly spiritual society where individuals deeply believe in voodoo and black magic, it may very well be possible that a combination of mild paralytic agents coupled with hypnotic suggestion might place someone in a state of stupor resembling that of a zombie.

Japanese researchers refer to three stages of fugu (tetrodotoxin) poisoning. The first is characterized by a progressive numbing sensation throughout the body and a loss of motor function, similar to falling into deep sleep. The second stage involves body paralysis, labored breathing, and a sharp drop in blood pressure. While all this is happening, the victim can see and hear what is going on around him. At the last stage, death comes as a result of acute respiratory failure. If the fugu eater has not consumed too much toxin, the last stage is avoided. However, the victim does remain in a state of suspended animation for an extended period of time—much like a Haitian zombie, only richer.

EVENT 19. THE QUICK AND THE DEAD

Escherichia coli bacteria were first described by the German pediatrician and bacteriologist Dr. Theodore Escherich, in an article he published in 1885 titled "The Intestine Bacteria of the Newborn Child and Infants."[44] These bacteria existed in great numbers in the intestine (colon), so he called them *Bacterium coli*. Years after this discovery, the bacteria were renamed *Escherichia coli* in his honor. For more than one hundred years, these microorganisms were not considered to be very harmful. However, because they were so common in the intestines and feces, they were used as an indicator of contamination in bodies of water into which sewage flowed. Similarly, in the food industry, regulators used the existence of *Escherichia coli* as an indicator of poor sanitation practices on the part of company employees.

The varieties of *E. coli* considered to be pathogenic to humans were those that caused diarrhea. The most common one was called enteropathogenic and was most often implicated in infant diarrhea—a condition that could end up being chronic unless great care was taken to ensure that the baby bottles, diapers, linens, and toys were kept scrupulously clean. These measures were (and are) necessary to prevent reinfection by passing or direct contact with a baby's feces. Two other types of pathogenic *E. coli* were known as enteroinvasive and enterotoxigenic forms.

Historically, the most well-known form of pathogenic *E. coli* is the enterotoxigenic type. It occurs most commonly in developing countries where sanitation remains at a very low level and is responsible for the range of diarrheal symptoms experienced by travelers with such fanciful names as Montezuma's Revenge, Delhi Belly, Rangoon Runs, Tokyo Trots, and the more generic Gringo Gallop.

Before going any further, it may be useful to provide a cursory explanation of how bacteria evolve certain pathogenic characteristics. Most of us are familiar with the concept of inheritance through genes—those small sections of a chromosome that carry the codes for particular characteristics. Unlike the cells of higher organisms that carry their chromosomes within a well-defined nucleus, bacterial cells usually contain a large circular chromosome that is not enclosed by a membrane of any sort and is free to move around within the cytoplasm. In addition, bacterial cells may contain several smaller circular strands of DNA called plasmids, which can operate independently from a microorganism's main chromosome.

A microbe's characteristics are defined by the DNA in both its large chromosome and its plasmids. Very often characteristics such as antibiotic resistance—a microorganism's ability to withstand the effects of antibiotics—are carried in plasmids. It is a quirk of nature that bacteria, which may not be related to one another, are able to share characteristics through a process of plasmid transfer. That is why antibiotic resistance can spread so quickly between various species of bacteria. Another way is through bacteriophage transfer.

A bacteriophage is a small virus that can infect bacteria. Since all viruses are essentially DNA, bacteriophages infect bacteria and incorporate their own DNA into that of the bacteria. The bacteriophage begins to replicate itself until the bacterial cell bursts and disperses a cloud of young new bacteriophages ready to infect a great many more bacteria. At times, these bacteriophages are able to incorporate the DNA from one bacterium and pass it on to others that they infect.

E. coli's prevalence in the colon stems from its basic ability to cling to the inner surface of the intestines, causing some of the lining cells to perish. This particular characteristic is carried in the bacteria's plasmids and can easily be transferred to other bacteria such as non-pathogenic *E. coli*. This results in a greater number of *E. coli* types that can cause occasional diarrhea.

In another case, enteroinvasive *E. coli* inherited the ability to actually invade the surface cells of the intestine by picking up genetic material from another bacterium called *Shigella flexneri*. Although they are from two completely different families of bacteria, both species produce the same symptoms, because they share identical pathogenicities. In this case, the bacteriophage passed on the DNA that coded for the deadly Shiga toxin, and thereby created a new superbug.

It is thought that this bacteriophage-moderated DNA transfer may have been accelerated by the use of antibiotics in cattle feed. However, this has not yet been proven with any certainty. What is certain is that *Escherichia coli* O157:H7 is one very deadly bacterium.

Our traditional perception of the quasi-benign nature of *E. coli* changed dramatically in the 1990s when the first highly publicized cases of enterohemorrhagic *E. coli* occurred.

It is thought that the *E. coli* O157:H7 originally evolved as early as 1955 because Hemolytic Uremic Syndrome—a typical characteristic of *E. coli* O157:H7—was first described by a Swiss pediatrician while examining a dairy-related outbreak. (Hemolytic Uremic Syndrome, or HUS, is characterized by sudden gastrointestinal bleeding, anemia, blood in the urine, and renal failure.) Another incident of *E. coli* occurred in 1975, when doctors took a stool sample from a California-based female naval officer who had a severe case of bloody diarrhea. They cultured a rare form of *E. coli* and sent it to the Centers for Disease Control and Prevention (CDC) in Atlanta, where it was promptly placed in storage. In December 1981, a severe outbreak of hemorrhagic diarrhea occurred in White City, Oregon. Local physicians were unable to identify the responsible organism and called Dr. Lee Riley, a California-based epidemiologist who was associated with the CDC. No specific microbial agent was immediately found, but shortly thereafter another outbreak occurred, this time in Michigan— and, as was the case in the Oregon outbreak, a McDonald's restaurant was implicated. By this time, Joy Wells, a microbiologist at the CDC, isolated *E. coli* O157:H7 from stool samples of the victims. However, it was not until two months later that investigators discovered the same *E. coli* O157:H7 in a processing plant that had supplied the suspicious burgers to McDonald's. It was then that Dr. Wells took it one step further and canvassed the thousands of *E. coli* samples maintained at the CDC and found the one that had been responsible for the hemorrhagic diarrhea episode that took place in 1975.

The scientists were finally onto something conclusive and in 1982 they published the results in the *New England Journal of Medicine*.[45]

When *E. coli* O157:H7 was first discovered, it was a true rarity among pathogenic bacteria because no one could accurately estimate the minimum infectious dose (the minimum number of organisms required to cause an infection). For most bacteria, the average infectious dose ranged from 100 to 1,000,000,000, however for *E. coli* O157:H7, its pathogenicity was so great that the ingestion of one single cell was thought to be sufficient to cause an infection. Even then, its true potential wasn't fully known because the outbreaks of it had been so limited.

A decade after the conclusive discovery of *E. coli* O157:H7 pathogenicity, I recall specifically bringing up the subject at an international meeting on food safety in Orlando, Florida.[46] I was so impressed with its high potential for infectivity as well as its severe symptoms that I felt obliged to ask one of the senior government speakers what the government was doing about *E. coli* O157:H7. The reply I got was that little was being done, since it was very uncommon and as a result was not considered to be a major problem. It was a very unsatisfying answer to be sure, but very few food-safety regulators understood the seriousness of the threat.

Exactly two months later, toward the end of December 1992, at the height of the Christmas holiday period, the Shiga hit the fan!

In early January 1993, a Seattle pediatrician noticed what he thought was an unusual spike in the number of children coming down with bloody diarrhea. He immediately alerted the Washington State health officials about a possible foodborne outbreak. He was absolutely right.

In less than a week, the health department staff successfully identified hamburgers contaminated with *E. coli* O157:H7 bacteria from the Jack in the Box restaurant chain as the cause of the outbreak. More than seventy Jack in the Box restaurants located in Washington, Nevada, California, and Idaho were involved in the outbreak and immediate recall.

Seven hundred people became very ill and four children died. The staff epidemiologists at the Centers for Disease Control and Prevention quickly concluded that the outbreak resulted from errors in meat processing at the plant that made the burgers in addition to improper cooking at the restaurants that served them.[47] Ultimately, this incident turned out to be a defining moment in the history of food safety in the United States.

This was certainly not the first large-scale foodborne disease outbreak to be recorded. More than ten years earlier in 1982, two large outbreaks of Norwalk gastroenteritis occurred in Minnesota. The first one involved three thousand cases and was related to eating bakery items with contaminated frosting; the second involved two thousand

cases and was associated with eating bad coleslaw. In 1988 a large outbreak of *Shigella sonnei* infections occurred among the unfortunate
individuals who ate what was supposed to be a healthy raw tofu salad
at an outdoor music festival in Michigan. In this outbreak, 3,175
people became ill; 117 cases were serious enough to require hospitalization. The Jack in the Box incident paled in comparison to the
national outbreak of *Salmonella enteritidis* infections from Schwan's
ice cream that occurred a year later, in which almost one-quarter of a
million people were infected.[48]

What made the Jack in the Box incident a watershed event was that
four children died an unusually cruel and agonizing death—from the
simple act of eating a hamburger. Hamburgers are the quintessential icon
of American fast food. There is no other food as ubiquitous throughout
America as the hamburger. By the time of the outbreak, McDonald's
alone had sold over eighty billion hamburgers around the world.

One of the saddest comments following the outbreak was made by
Michael Nole of Tacoma, the father of one of the victims. "I don't care
how long I live, I will never believe that my son died from eating a
cheeseburger. Never."[49] His son, Michael James, died at Children's
Hospital and Medical Center in Tacoma. He died from complications
resulting from Hemolytic Uremic Syndrome, or HUS—a condition in
which platelets start to clump within the kidney's tiny blood vessels,
resulting in reduced blood flow and eventual kidney failure. The partial blockage of the blood vessels also leads to destruction of red cells.
Michael was twenty-five months old.

Although it is unusual to include such a long quote from another
source, I found the testimony of Michael's mother so touching that I
have reproduced it in large part from the S.T.O.P. Web site.

> My son had bouts of diarrhea, which rapidly became runny, painful
> and eventually bloody . . . and later all blood.
>
> He was admitted to Mary Bridge Children's Hospital in Tacoma,
> Washington. I had no idea what was soon to follow.

The bloody diarrhea continued throughout the night, every 3–5 minutes with screams of pain and terror with each one. We went through a diaper with each one because the blood burned his skin.

In the morning, he was transferred to the pediatric I.C.U. unit. Unknown to us, there were already children there with *E. coli* O157:H7.

By this time his kidneys had shut down and he was becoming very lethargic, his abdomen began to swell to an unbelievable size. He had hemorrhoids and was unable to eat or urinate.

I remember the last time my husband and I saw our son responding and sitting up with our help. Due to his swollen tummy and tubes in his arms, he ate an orange popsicle and I kept trying to tell myself he was going to be okay.

Dialysis was needed and the decision was made to transport him to a children's hospital in Seattle that had the machines for this purpose.

Before they transported him I had asked to rock him in my arms in a chair next to his bed. With the help of 3 nurses and his physician, they carried him over to me with all of his tubes, IV's and other monitoring devices and set him in my arms.

I rocked him and sang our favorite songs together. One of our favorites was "Jesus Loves Me." To this day, I cannot bear to hear this song.

This was the last time I held my baby in my arms.

He was transported to Children's Hospital in Seattle, I rode in the ambulance with him and two other transport nurses. We made the hour trip in 22 minutes. . . .

Michael had dialysis one or two times a day. There were so many other children arriving daily that needed dialysis that the machines were becoming very popular. Nurses, physicians and all other specialists were working around the clock, many sleeping at the hospital to provide the best possible care for our children.

As Michael's meds increased and tried to help his pains, things got even worse.

The physicians thought we might lose him at several different times, and several times we were rushed in to say our last good-byes and prayers. This was so very painful.

As our family members started to arrive to kiss his cheek and stroke his golden hair and say prayers I just sat back in complete helplessness, thinking "I'm his mommy . . . why can't I fix this? Make everything better? Trade him places?" This was such a hopeless, powerless feeling. After physicians noted he had red patches on his tummy, they thought something might have burst inside him. The suggestion was made to rush him into surgery to see if they could stop or identify the internal bleeding.

Papers were signed and we kissed him good-bye one more time in the hallway on his way to surgery.

I cannot remember how long it took . . . 1, 2, 3, hours, seemed like 2 days.

When he returned they said they "lost" him once during surgery but were able to revive him.

When we were allowed to go in to see him he had an incision from his neck to his groin area. This was so difficult to see.

He did not do well after this, he opened his eyes once, and we were able to see the blue of his eyes and barely a twinkle. I told him he was mommies big boy and that I would love him forever and someday would be with him forever in heaven. My husband and I spent several hours with him before he died. The nurses gave me a lock of his golden hair to cherish.

I left the hospital with his blanket, shoes, choo-choo train, sweats I
made for him, and a bag of toys.[50]

As his father said, all Michael did was eat a cheeseburger.

Based on documents filed in the US District Court in Seattle, the
Jack in the Box restaurant chain had made a decision to cook their hamburger patties at a temperature below that recommended by state regulations (155°F). Had they cooked the burgers at the recommended temperature, in all likelihood, the *E. coli* O157:H7 that contaminated the
meat would have been killed. The Jack in the Box restaurant chain purchased this batch of frozen hamburger patties from Vons Companies
Inc. The Jack in the Box parent company Foodmaker blamed and eventually sued Vons, claiming that it was responsible for the outbreak.

The Jack in the Box outbreak in 1993 made *E. coli* O157:H7 a
household word. The devastation it brought to families whose children
died or ended up with lifelong disabilities served as a rude wake-up
call to a nation that took the safety of its favorite food for granted.

No sooner had the Jack in the Box outbreak subsided than another
national outbreak hit the press. This time, it was an upscale unpas-
teurized apple juice that carried the deadly *E. coli* O157:H7 bacteria.
While it wasn't difficult to understand how ground-up hamburger
could be contaminated, how was it possible that apple juice could
carry the same bacteria?

The stream of unanswered questions began to mount up. What
were we doing to allow such things to happen? What changes had been
made to standard quality-control procedures? If it could happen in
products differing as widely as hamburger and apple juice, where
might it strike next? Were the laws we were working under no longer
sufficient to deal with this new threat? The increasing number of negative articles in the media dictated that some radical changes had to be
made before the industry could restore the consumer's confidence in
the food supply.

The National Food Safety Initiative began with President Bill
Clinton's radio address in January 1997: "We have built a solid founda-

tion for the health of America's families. But clearly we must do more. No parent should have to think twice about the juice they pour their children at breakfast, or a hamburger ordered during dinner out."[51]

The goal of the initiative was to identify all possible contamination points along the farm-to-table continuum and implement process controls for preventing problems that might affect our nation's food supply.

For the first time, representatives from Agriculture, Health and Human Services, the Food and Drug Administration, the Centers for Disease Control and Prevention, the Department of Defense, the Environmental Protection Agency, the Council of State and Territorial Epidemiologists, the Association of Food and Drug Officials, the Association of Public Health Laboratories, the National Association of City and County Health Officers, the Association of State and Territorial Health Officials, and the National Association of State Departments of Agriculture were put together to solve the problem. No one was to be left out.

The resulting Farm to Table approach clearly recognized that food safety began at the production level and included all the steps in the process from the farm to the ultimate consumer's table. Likewise, the key government agencies recognized the importance of a seamless interagency approach to food-safety problems.

In order to test how effectively interagency cooperation worked, a joint program was set up to develop a method for the rapid detection of *E. coli* O157:H7. The Centers for Disease Control and Prevention published a list of all those diseases that could be transmitted by the food supply.[52] Various state public health agencies began to publish their own food-safety initiatives.

In 2006 there was a national *E. coli* O157:H7 outbreak, this time the culprit was spinach. The increasing number of vegetables contaminated with animal pathogens highlighted the growing problems of industrial-scale agricultural production. In this case, cattle ranching operations were located upstream from large vegetable cultivation areas. Runoff containing infected animal waste made its way from the beef production operation to the spinach fields, resulting in major *E. coli* contamination. No doubt, this will result in truly major changes to the future of adjacent animal and vegetable agricultural production.

The National Food Safety Initiative began an overhaul of food-safety programs that continues to the present. These changes have brought about the most integrated food safety and surveillance systems in the world, resulting in one of the world's safest food supplies.

And it all started with Jack in the Box.

EVENT 20. BIOTERRORISM AND THE FOOD SUPPLY

Although I was originally reluctant to focus on bioterrorism in this book, it would not be appropriate to avoid the subject in today's post-9/11 world. We all must eat to survive, and food or beverages are natural vehicles to deliver the threat of bioterrorism.

The term *terrorism* generally refers to premeditated and politically motivated violence against civilian targets by groups, usually with the intent to gain influence. The National Security Institute defines *terrorism* as the use of force or violence against persons or property in violation of the criminal laws of the United States for purposes of intimidation, coercion, or ransom.

Nonetheless, there is no universally accepted definition of bioterrorism. In the most general terms, bioterrorism involves the actual or threatened use of biological agents by individuals or groups that are motivated by political, economic, social, ecological, religious, or other ideological goals. Most definitions of terrorism focus on the aim of intimidating governments or societies, but even that is not always the case.

Some terrorists are attracted to any weapons that can cause massive casualties, simply because they want to cause death on an unprecedented scale. Individuals or groups with apocalyptic visions and/or a desire to exact revenge for a perceived wrong want to kill as many people as possible. In the past, terrorists used violence as a means to an end, but today we are seeing more and more terrorists for whom murder and violence is the desired end.

The biological agents commonly used in bioterrorism are organisms or their toxins that are effective in harming people, animals, or plants. Chemical agents, on the other hand, are poisonous substances from humanmade materials, but they are sometimes included in the bioterrorism literature.

There are literally hundreds of organisms that can do us harm, including bacteria, viruses, fungi, and parasites. Among the pathogens often considered as possible bioterror agents are *Bacillus anthracis*, the anthrax bacteria, and *Yersinia pestis*, the bacteria that caused the Black Plague. Other frightening organisms include *Mycobacterium leprae*, the bacteria responsible for leprosy, and *Wuchereria bancrofti*, the microscopic filarial worm that causes elephantiasis—both diseases that result in such dreadful disfigurations they would easily serve to terrorize.

The poisonous toxins produced by living organisms include those derived from plants, animals, and microorganisms. Among the best known are the deadly botulinum toxin from the bacteria *Clostridium botulinum*; ricin, a toxin extracted from castor beans; and tetrodotoxin from fugu fish. Of course, there are hundreds of others derived from roots, beans, flowers, mushrooms, sea creatures, snakes, frogs, not to mention other microorganisms. There is no scarcity of biological sources from which to derive fatal toxins.

Although it is a little more difficult to gain access to purified biological agents than it was in the very recent past, it is not impossible. All varieties of organisms, including some very pathogenic ones, are stored in academic or commercial culture collections in various countries around the world and, in the past, have served as preferred sources of materials for terrorists. Anyone who can masquerade as a researcher can usually gain access to these organisms. Requirements for access in certain countries have recently been tightened, but these organisms are available for purchase in other countries. Alternatively, one need only recruit a poorly paid or ideologically motivated technician who has access to these organisms. In the recent past, the legal or quasi-legal acquisition of pathogenic biological agents has proven to be relatively easy.

Of course, for those who cannot or will not follow the legal or quasi-legal path, then outright theft is the next best approach. While laboratories in developed countries may have strict security, this is definitely not the case in developing countries where pathogenic organisms may simply be stored in a refrigerator that many people have access to without any security at all. In some cases there is no need to achieve your means with stealth and glass cutters, you can simply walk in during the daytime and pinch a test tube or a Petri dish right out of the departmental fridge.

If all else fails, there is the possibility of culturing pathogenic organisms from scratch from any number of sources—the soil, human or animal waste, garbage, or any other putrefying mess. Pathogens exist everywhere. The problem with this final approach is that you really have to know what you're doing, and this knowledge is usually beyond the abilities of most terrorists—so far.

I have a particular interest in bioterrorism because one of the first recorded cases in North America involved the university department where I originally intended to do my postgraduate work. Fascinated by the amazing range of invertebrate creatures and inspired by the thought of curing some of the most ghastly diseases afflicting people in the developing world, I applied and was accepted into the department of parasitology at McGill University's Macdonald College campus in Ste. Anne de Bellevue, Quebec, in 1968. Several weeks before starting courses, my supervisor-to-be accepted an opportunity to do an overseas sabbatical, and I thought it best to do my graduate work at another university where I would be under the close supervision of a full-time mentor.

A little more than a year later, one of the graduate students in Macdonald's department of parasitology, Eric Kranz, a twenty-three-year-old from New York City, was having problems with his roommates. He reportedly wasn't paying his share of the rent, and on January 24, 1970, he was told to leave the Maple Avenue boardinghouse in Ste.

Anne de Bellevue, the closest town to the Macdonald campus. He refused to leave immediately, and was asked to leave again in early February. This time Kranz left.

On February 10, one of the other students suddenly became violently ill and was admitted to the hospital for observation. Shortly thereafter, the other boardinghouse students became sick. Hospital staff members were baffled and at first thought it was a bad case of pneumonia. The condition of one of the students quickly deteriorated to a point where he had to be placed in an intensive care unit under artificial respiration.

Later, Dr. Eugene Meerovitch of Macdonald's department of parasitology, whom I remember as having terribly fatigue-ringed eyes from spending so much time looking into microscopes, identified worms in the sputum samples from the students. Further analysis confirmed that the worms were the species *Ascaris suum*—a parasite found not in humans but in pigs! Consultations with Walter Reed Army Hospital confirmed that such a parasitic infection had never been detected in humans. The ensuing investigation in Quebec seemed to indicate that the students may have eaten contaminated food on January 29, five days after they told their roommate Kranz to leave.[53]

Ascaris suum worms live as adults in the intestines of infected pigs, where the females can grow to a length of fifteen inches. A gravid female may produce up to two hundred thousand eggs per day, which are shed out with the feces. If they are ingested, the eggs hatch two to three weeks later. The tiny worms (about 1/100th of an inch long) burrow through the intestinal mucosa and are carried by the bloodstream through the liver and into the blood spaces of the lungs. The larvae mature further in the lungs (ten to fourteen days), where they cause the pneumonia-like symptoms. They can be coughed up with the sputum, which is how Meerovitch identified them. The worms are then swallowed and, upon reaching the small intestine, they develop into adult worms. An excellent representation of the *Ascaris* life cycle is shown in the accompanying CDC representation.[54]

As soon as it was suspected that the sick students had ingested parasite eggs with their food, the police were called in and warrants were sworn out against Eric Kranz for attempted murder. But Kranz was nowhere to be found.[55]

As soon as he learned that one of his fellow roommates got ill, Kranz decided to leave Canada. On February 14, he fled to New York. New York police cooperated in the investigation and questioned Kranz's parents, but they said they had not seen him in several years. Two weeks later, on March 1, Kranz landed in Mexico City and went to the suburb of Del Valle, but soon headed out to destinations unknown, possibly Veracruz.[56]

At high noon on Monday, March 9, Eric Kranz walked into Quebec provincial police headquarters in Montreal with his lawyer.[57] Apparently, the police had been in contact with Kranz's lawyer during the previous week. (It still baffles me that Kranz had the means to escape to New York and Mexico and to hire a costly criminal lawyer, but he supposedly could not pay his share of the boardinghouse rent.)

Just prior to Kranz's return to Canada, the four students that were poisoned recovered sufficiently to be released from hospital. This may have had an impact upon Kranz's decision to return to Canada to face trial.

Kranz was held without bail until March 17, when the judge set his bail at $15,000, which was promptly made by his father, a New York dentist. A day later, Kranz was sent to trial on four charges of attempted murder.[58] Unfortunately, the story ends there since I have not been able to learn the decision of the court.

Thus, one of the first cases of bioterrorism in North America faded from view.

While the Eric Kranz case was considered to be one of the first in North America to use a biological weapon, the FBI considers the next case to be the first such case to occur on US soil. It involved the use of biological agents by a religious cult, the Rajneeshees, in a small town in Oregon called The Dalles. When this case was over, almost eight hundred people had been poisoned, the cult had escaped to more sympathetic environs, and the town's economy was left in shambles. Not bad for a movement that extolled peace and religious tolerance.

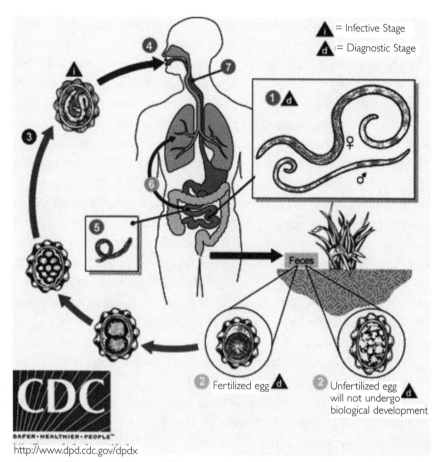

= Infective Stage

= Diagnostic Stage

Fertilized egg

Unfertilized egg will not undergo biological development

CDC
SAFER·HEALTHIER·PEOPLE™
http://www.dpd.cdc.gov/dpdx

Ascaris life cycle, from Centers for Disease Control and Prevention, http://www.dpd.cdc.gov/dpdx/html/ImageLibrary/Ascariasis_il.asp?body=A-F/Ascariasis/body_Ascariasis_il11.htm (accessed August 24, 2006).

The history of Rajneeshism is a long and distasteful one. The founder, guru Bhagwan Shree Rajneesh, was a complex man who may have originally started out with good intentions but ultimately drifted to the dark side in a desire to acquire riches and enjoy the lifestyle of the wealthy. Rajneesh was born on December 11, 1931, in the town of Kuchwada in Madya Pradesh, India's Tiger State. When his childhood girlfriend died in 1947, he went into a deep depression. After coming out of it, he considered himself an "enlightened" man.[59] He graduated from high school in 1951 and began to study philosophy at college, but had a great deal of difficulty keeping his mental faculties intact. He tried to manage this problem with steady meditation.

He eventually graduated from college in 1955 with an MA in philosophy and went on to become an assistant professor at the University of Jabalpur in 1960. Rajneesh started giving public lectures about the divine energy of sex. Not surprisingly, this subject attracted a great many followers. He developed a new method of meditation in which worshipers began by jumping around and shouting whatever came into their minds. The idea was to put yourself into a state of hyperventilation, from which you would "see the light," if you didn't pass out first.

By the fall of 1970, he started the Neo-Sannyas International Movement and in the following year he changed his name to Bhagwan (Blessed One) Shree Rajneesh. The Blessed One started to gain a great many Western followers.

He set up his first ashram in the city of Poona, India, with a few fellow Indian disciples. Rajneesh steadily became more well known, and by 1976, he was one of the main attractions on the guru travel circuit frequented by many Westerners searching for a greater meaning in their lives. As a result of the cult's beliefs, it encountered opposition in the larger Indian society, so the Bhagwan decided to move his ashram to a new location. One of his more aggressive followers, Ma Anand Sheela, an Indian woman who attended a university in the United States, convinced Rajneesh to move his operation to the United States in 1981. The pickings were much better in the United States, and, besides, by this time, the majority of the Rajneeshees were Westerners.

In short order, Sheela bought a sixty-four-thousand-acre Oregon property known as the Big Muddy Ranch for $5.6 million, even though it was evaluated for tax purposes at only $200,000. A large part of the ranch was located in Wasco County, a rural area with a population of about twenty thousand. The seat of Wasco County was a small town called The Dalles, which had a population of around ten thousand people. Little did these townsfolk know what was about to descend upon them.

After the Rajneeshees purchased the Big Muddy Ranch, they set about building their new ashram. Under Ma Anand Sheela's continually growing influence, the focus of the Rajneeshees shifted from leading a highly spiritual life to making money. There was a great pressure to work and an even greater pressure to transfer all their earnings to the ashram. To reflect their growing wealth, Rajneesh, the Blessed One, began driving around the commune in one of his growing fleet of Rolls Royce automobiles.

Right from the start, trouble began to brew between the ashram and Wasco County. The most contentious problems between the Rajneeshees and the surrounding community resulted from Oregon's tough land use laws, which greatly limited development in rural areas—not a very convenient situation for an ambitious ashram. In order to continue their expansion of Rajneeshpuram (the new name of their ashram), the cult decided to work around the laws. Using the state's own liberal voter registration laws, they decided to grab control of a nearby town of only forty residents called Antelope. They accomplished this by building several housing units to supplement the ones on the ashram and then proposing to build a large office facility and several other new buildings there. The horrified Antelope city council refused to give them building permits on the grounds that there was not enough water to support all this new construction.

The Rajneeshees decided to pursue legal action and eventually were permitted to develop their current properties, but they were not allowed any future development. The agreement did not last long, and the irrepressible Rajneeshees took full control of the city council, running out the remaining older residents. It is safe to say that this was the turning point in relations between the Rajneeshees and the other inhabitants of Wasco County, simply because it offended many people who normally would not have given the group a second thought. The Rajneeshees then took over the Antelope school board and became known in the greater Oregon political scene as a genuine threat to rural community life.

By the beginning of 1984, the cult was under considerable pressure from the US attorney's office in Portland. The office started an immigration investigation that could have led to the deportation of many Rajneeshees, including the Bhagwan. Even the state's attorney general was investigating the legal status of Rajneeshpuram.

Tensions were growing in response to all the legal actions and a number of inflammatory television appearances by Sheela. By 1984 the ashram had acquired an arsenal of semiautomatic weapons and handguns for its new police force, known as the Peace Force. As a result of Sheela's manipulations, the ashram started to take on characteristics of George Orwell's *Animal Farm*. All power may have derived from the Bhagwan's authority, but he had no involvement in the daily operations of the organization other than his daily Rolls Royce cruise through the ashram. Sheela ran the cult, controlled the finances, and directed all the operations of Rajneeshpuram through her small inner circle of trusted women, referred to as the "moms."

Because Sheela was accountable only to the Blessed One, everyone had to toe the line or risk being "turfed out" of Rajneeshpuram. The ashram became more militant and built a large fence around the Bhagwan's residence, complete with sentry posts. One member of the ashram told of a conversation she had with one of the armed sentries, who had previously been a close friend of hers. She asked why the man's attitude toward her had grown so distant. He replied, "Sheela's orders, she says it isn't good to get friendly with people you might have to shoot."[60] The ashram had made the transition from spirituality and enlightenment to greed and violence.

Sheela lost patience and, in consort with her inner circle, decided that the Wasco County Court was a problem that had to be dealt with. The county court controlled the permits that the Rajneeshees needed and the court's growing truculence was proving to be a major impediment to the cult's ambitions.

The Wasco County Court was made up of three elected commissioners. As it happened, two of them were up for reelection in November 1984. Sheela, with the Bhagwan's approval, decided to gain control of the Wasco County Court by manipulating the election. She did this by bringing thousands of homeless people to Rajneeshpuram. Once they were considered to be local residents, they would be immediately eligible to vote in the November election. In order to put the finishing touches to this plan, Sheela came up with an additional strategy. To ensure victory for the Rajneeshees, Sheela decided to poison the local water supply in order to make the Wasco County voters so sick they wouldn't be able to vote.

Thus was hatched the first plan for large-scale bioterrorism in the United States.

As a result of the FBI investigation that followed the incident, we are able to learn a great deal about how the Rajneeshees executed the plan to use biological agents against the local residents. Much of the information came from Krishna Diva (David Berry Knapp)—the former mayor of Rajneeshpuram—and was expertly documented by Dr. Seth Carus in his working paper "Bioterrorism and Biocrimes."[61]

According to the testimony of Krishna Diva, Sheela hatched the idea and, together with her close associate Ma Anand Puja, began looking into the possibility of using biological agents in a serious way.

Ma Anand Puja (Dianne Onang) is considered to be the person most directly involved in obtaining and developing the biological agents used by the Rajneeshees. Born in the Philippines and brought up in California, Ma Anand Puja took up nursing and was registered in 1997. She then left the United States to work in clinics throughout her native Philippines and Indonesia. She traveled to India and, after first hearing the Bhagwan speak, decided to join his ashram in Poona. Because of her background, she became the director of the ashram's health center and soon became very tight with Sheela.

Once the cult moved to the United States, Puja had full control over all of Rajneeshpuram's medical facilities. However, her real power, which extended far beyond the medical arena, came from her close association with Sheela. Her tyrannical behavior made her unpopular with other ashram members, who sometimes referred to her as "Dr. Mengele" (the infamous Nazi doctor). In subsequent interrogations, Krishna Diva described Puja as someone who delighted in death and savored the idea of carrying out plots involving poisons. He even suggested that some people thought that Puja was involved in the mysterious death of Sheela's first husband in 1980.

In preparing to execute Sheela's plans, Puja looked at several different biological agents to make people sick. To avoid suspicion, she elected to use an organism that is commonly found in cases of food poisoning, *Salmonella typhimurium*. Puja also considered several other biological agents, including *Salmonella typhi*, the organism that causes typhoid fever. Puja liked the idea of using typhoid bacteria, because it was likely to cause several weeks of debilitating fever. Fortunately, because of the greater risk involved in using it—the ashram members themselves could also become infected—this organism was eventually abandoned.

Based on further testimony from Krishna Diva, it appears that Puja was seriously contemplating infecting people with the AIDS virus. Apparently, she purchased a freeze-dried sample of the virus specifically for that purpose. But other than an unconfirmed report that Puja deliberately infected one individual with HIV, there is no indication that this lethal organism was used.

As unbelievable as it may sound, the Rajneeshees obtained their pathogenic strain of *Salmonella typhimurium* simply by ordering it from a commercial supplier. The cultures are delivered as purified disks containing the freeze-dried bacteria. It is a simple matter to grow these in sterile culture media if you have the required equipment— which is also easy to obtain. It appears that the cultures of *S. typhimurium* were produced in a secret laboratory located directly on the grounds of Rajneeshpuram, the ashram of enlightenment.

Everything was now in place for Sheela and her cohorts to start doing their dirty work. The first opportunity came on August 29, 1984, when three of the Wasco County commissioners came to Rajneeshpuram for a routine fact-finding visit. Two of the commissioners, Judge William Hulse and Commissioner Ray Matthew, were kindly offered glasses of water, which the Rajneeshees had previously conta-

minated with *S. typhimurium*. Both men became very sick, and Judge
Hulse ended up in the hospital.

Apparently, the Rajneeshees tried going after a larger swath of
people at the Wasco County Courthouse by spreading some of the
liquid *S. typhimurium* culture throughout the building on doorknobs
and flush knobs of toilets, but this did not have the desired effect, since
no one became ill. It is likely that the organisms did not survive when
exposed to the air and dried slowly. While it is possible that some
organisms survived and cross-contaminated the hands of individuals,
they could have been washed off or they may not have constituted a
sufficient dose to cause an incident.

Armed with the knowledge that the best way to make people sick
was to contaminate the foods they were eating and drinking, the cult
went about sprinkling liquid culture on salads at a local supermarket
with the goal of giving the local people the "runs." It is not known
what the effects of these small individual tests were, but regardless of
the outcome, by early September 1984, Sheela and her merry band of
poisoners were now ready to do some serious testing.

Armed with what was obviously a considerable amount of *S.
typhimurium*, the cult members began pouring vials of culture into
food products at various restaurants throughout The Dalles. Their
favorite targets were the attractive salad bars found in so many restaurants. People naturally gravitate to the salad bar because of the variety
of products and its reputation for being healthy. Dressed in "civilian"
clothes rather than their traditional orange ashram garb, the
Rajneeshees added their poisonous *S. typhimurium* brew to the salads,
the salad dressings, and other condiments at the salad bar. Not satisfied with that, they added it to the coffee creamers as well. They were
successful beyond their wildest dreams!

In a publication titled "A Large Community Outbreak of Salmo-
nellosis Caused by Intentional Contamination of Restaurant Salad
Bars," staff members of the National Center for Infectious Diseases and
Epidemiology at the Centers for Disease Control and Prevention in
Atlanta describe how 751 people became ill after eating at salad bars in

several restaurants.[62] The investigators had systematically ruled out all the possibilities of accidental contamination occurring as a result of poor practices or due to unhygienic sanitation habits on the part of employees at the various restaurants. The inescapable conclusion was that the poisonings were the result of a number of deliberate acts. There is little doubt that the actual number of victims was considerably higher than the 751 reported because The Dalles is located by an interstate highway and any number of unsuspecting travelers passing through town may have been infected, but as is often the case in foodborne disease outbreaks, their cases would not have been reported.

After their successes at the restaurants, the Rajneeshees ceased their attacks. The enormous publicity generated by the epidemic made it evident that their plot to poison the water supply would fail. The Rajneeshees abandoned their efforts to take over Wasco County.

Bioterrorism was initially considered only a remote explanation for the outbreak when public health officials were first investigating the case. In 1984 no one imagined anyone could be mad enough to do such a thing. It was only after the FBI began investigating the cult for other criminal violations that the source of the attack surfaced. A vial of *S. Typhimurium*, identical to the particular strain responsible for the outbreak, was found in the laboratory at Rajneeshpuram. Then, members of the ashram began spilling the beans. It was not long before they admitted to contaminating the salad bars with *Salmonella* and planning to contaminate the city's water supply.

In November hearings were held on the use of federal land in and around the ashram by the Rajneeshees, and bills were introduced to repeal the charter of Rajneeshpuram. In March of 1985, the state superintendent of schools threatened to cut off aid to the Rajneeshee school.

The Rajneeshees succeeded no further in their political ambitions. Federal investigations into their operations progressed. Even though Sheela had destroyed a great deal of information, there was enough evidence for a federal grand jury to issue a thirty-five-count indictment charging the Bhagwan, Sheela, and six others with conspiracy to evade the immigration laws.[63]

The Blessed One attempted to flee from the law, but his private jet was intercepted in North Carolina, where he was seized and incarcerated. Despite his lawyer's pleas that the Bhagwan was too ill to be kept in jail, he was soon returned to Oregon. He pled guilty to concealing his intent to remain in the United States and lying to immigration officials in 1981. He agreed to pay $400,000 in fines and court costs—not a particularly difficult setback, since he was rolling in money. He was also handed a ten-year suspended prison sentence and ordered to leave the country within five days.

Sheela did manage to flee the country but was soon arrested in Germany. She was returned for trial in the United States and indicted on charges of attempted murder, conspiracy to commit murder, assault, wiretapping, arson, burglary, and the poisoning of two county commissioners—not bad for the manager of a commune devoted to love and revelation. She was fined almost $500,000 and ordered to give up her permanent resident status in the United States. She was also given concurrent prison terms but, incredibly, was released for good behavior after serving only two and a half years of her sentence in a federal medium-security prison. She eventually ended up in Basel, Switzerland, and opened up two nursing homes there. God bless the Swiss and their confidential banking system!

With the downturn in the fortunes of the Rajneeshee ashram, the world's largest fleet of Rolls Royces was suddenly put up for sale. However, it did not take long for the Bhagwan's ninety Rolls Royces, some painted in psychedelic colors, to be sold—thirty apparently went to a Middle Eastern buyer.

The Bhagwan left the United States for refuge in the Himalayas. He was not well received by the Indian public. He tried to reestablish his community but was met with hostility and opposition. He then went to Uruguay on the condition that he did not indulge in public criticism. He returned to Poona in 1990 and died there at the age of fifty-nine.

EVENT 21. THE POLITICS OF POISON

And forth he goes—no longer he would tarry—
Into the town unto a 'pothecary
And prayed him that he woulde sell
Some poison, that he might his rattes quell . . .
From the "Pardoner's Tale," in *The Canterbury Tales*,
Geoffrey Chaucer, 1343–1400

The use of poison to get rid of one's enemies dates as far back as written history. The first accounts were deciphered from tablets of the Sumerians of Mesopotamia (Iraq). The earliest known deity associated with poisoning was Gula, the Mistress of Charms and Spells or the Controller of Noxious Poisons. She is described on a cuneiform tablet purportedly written about 1400 BCE as:

Gula, the woman, the mighty one, the prince of all women.
His seed with a poison not curable
Without issue; in his body may she place
All the days of his life,
Blood and pus like water may he pour forth.

Poison was often referred to as the "coward's weapon" because its use is so premeditated, cold-blooded, and sneaky. Even more offensive, the poisoner knows that the victim is likely to experience prolonged suffering.

Despite its distasteful reputation, poisoning became so common throughout the ancient Roman Empire that a gathering of Roman jurists declared, "Armis bella non venensis geri," which roughly translates to "War should be fought with weapons, not poison."

Throughout the centuries, the rich and powerful employed tasters as a precaution against being poisoned—and for good reason. Political leaders and royalty have been favorite targets of the poisoner's art for millennia.

During the sixteenth century, both King Henry VIII and Queen Elizabeth lived in fear of being assassinated by poison. It was believed that Anne Boleyn had tried to poison Henry. Upon hearing this, the young Prince Henry supposedly "burst into tears saying that he and his sister, the Princess Mary, might thank God for having escaped from the hand of that accursed and venomous harlot who had intended to poison them."[64]

The tradition of using poison to assassinate political rivals or to eliminate dissidents has continued unabated to modern times. It is a strange tool for politicians and officials to use. Although it may be an efficient means of getting rid of enemies, poisoning, regardless of its sophistication, is often discovered. The incident thus gains far more notoriety than other methods, and the final outcome usually backfires.

Three recent incidents highlight examples of the use of poison for the purpose of political assassination.

The Georgi Markov Incident

Year	Victim	Poison	Location
1978	Georgi Markov	Ricin	London

Georgi Ivanov Markov was born in 1929, in Sofia, Bulgaria. Although he was trained as a chemical engineer, he started writing short stories after being hospitalized by an extended bout of tuberculosis. The quality of his work improved to the point where his 1962 novel, *Men*, won the Bulgarian Writers Annual Award. As his reputation grew, both he and his work came under the close scrutiny of the communist censors. Because his writing had become so popular, the communist leader Todor Zhivkov tried to intimidate Markov into serving his regime, but Markov didn't budge. His career took a decided turn for the worse when his 1969 play, *The Man Who Was Me*, was shown before an audience that included several Communist Party officials. They were not pleased, and all further performances of the play were cancelled. A close friend quietly warned Markov that he should leave Bulgaria. This time Markov listened and decided to head out for better climes.

After spending two years in Italy, Georgi Markov decided to move to England. In 1972 he started working for the BBC and became a freelance scriptwriter for Radio Free Europe, based in Munich, Germany. Because of his outspoken criticism of the Bulgarian government, all his written works were removed from Bulgarian bookshelves, and he was placed on trial and sentenced (in absentia) to six years and six months in prison for his defection. The Bulgarian Secret Service (the same organization allegedly involved in the attempted assassination of Pope John Paul) started a file on Markov.

Nevertheless, Markov continued his strong public criticism of Bulgaria's communist government and, in particular, its leader, Todor Zhivkov. Unfortunately, these personal attacks against Zhivkov, the Communist Party strongman, made Georgi Ivanov Markov a marked man. In July 1977, party boss Zhivkov signed a politburo decree stating, "All measures should be used to neutralize enemy émigrés." And Georgi Markov topped the enemies list.

On September 7, 1978, which also happened to be Zhivkov's birthday, the assassin sent to kill Bulgaria's most famous dissident struck. Markov parked his car below Waterloo Bridge and went up the stairs to join the queue at a bus stop. He felt a sharp jab in his right thigh and turned around quickly to see a man stooping down to pick up an umbrella he had apparently dropped. The man mumbled an apology and quickly walked away.

Markov immediately felt a stinging sensation in the back of his right leg, but despite the pain he continued on his way to work. When he arrived at the office of the BBC World Service, he went to the washroom. He looked at his leg and saw a small red spot that looked like a hive. The pain persisted, so he mentioned the incident to one of his colleagues. Later that evening, Markov developed a high fever and was taken to a hospital, where he was treated for blood poisoning. Unfortunately, the doctors did not have any clue as to what they were dealing with. Markov quickly went into shock and, after three days of utter agony, died.

Due to the statements Markov made to doctors concerning his suspicion that he was poisoned, Scotland Yard ordered a thorough forensic autopsy of Markov's body. The first thing that was noticed was that his lungs were full of fluid and his liver showed signs of acute blood poisoning. He had small hemorrhages all over his intestines, lymph nodes, and heart. And his white blood cell count was extremely high. Tissue was cut from around the puncture wound on Markov's right thigh and sent to the Chemical Defense Laboratory at Porton Down. There, almost by accident, they discovered a tiny metal pellet—a jeweler's watch bearing—just a little larger than the period at the end of this sentence.

The pellet measured 1.52 millimeters in diameter and was composed of 90 percent platinum and 10 percent iridium. It had two incredibly small cylinders with 0.35-millimeter diameters drilled through it in the shape of an X. The chemical experts found traces of ricin toxin in the X-shaped cavity. There was no known antidote to ricin poisoning. Markov had been a dead man while still standing and waiting for the bus.

Ricin is a toxin obtained from castor beans—more specifically, from the waste material left over from edible castor oil production. It has a structure similar to the botulinum toxin and works by entering the cells and shutting down protein synthesis. Without the required proteins, the cells die. Ricin is extremely toxic, with far less than a single milligram sufficient to kill a person. Because of its availability and lethality, ricin has long been considered as an ideal agent for biological warfare or bioterrorism.

In January 1979, after several months of investigation, the coroner's court in London ruled that Markov had been killed by 450 micrograms of lethal ricin toxin, contained in a miniature pellet injected with the aid of a specially designed umbrella that had been plunged into Markov's right thigh.

Despite the collapse of the Soviet Union, details of Markov's assassination and the link between the Bulgarian Secret Service and the Soviet KGB—which were thought to have supplied the toxin, the pellet, and the umbrella—remain hidden. The epitaph on Georgi

Markov's gravestone says it simply and elegantly: he died in the "cause of freedom."

The Viktor Yushchenko Incident

Year	Victim	Poison	Location
2004	Viktor Yushchenko	Dioxin	Kiev

Viktor Yushchenko was born on February 23, 1954, in Khoruzhivka, a small village in northern Ukraine. Both his parents were teachers. After graduating from the Ternopil Institute of Finance and Economics, he began his career as an accountant. He joined the banking system in 1976 and became deputy director for agricultural crediting at the Ukrainian office of the USSR State Bank in 1983. He further advanced to the position of vice chairman of the nonstate-run bank Ukraina, which specialized in agribusiness. Eventually, he was endorsed by parliament and appointed head of the Ukraine's Central Bank—the same year he completed his doctoral thesis and was awarded a Doctor of Economics degree.

In a surprise move, Ukrainian president Leonid Kuchma appointed Yushchenko to the post of prime minister in 1999. In 2001 Yushchenko was relieved of his power through a communist-inspired vote of no confidence. He immediately took over the leadership of the liberal opposition coalition known as Our Ukraine.

In the presidential elections of 2004, later to become known as the Ukraine's Orange Revolution, Yushchenko, considered to be pro-Western and a strong supporter of privatization, soon became the front runner. His opposing candidate, Viktor Yanukovych, was the favorite of both Leonid Kuchma and the man behind the scene, Russian president and former KGB officer Vladimir Putin.

On September 5, 2004, Viktor Yushchenko went to a dinner with heads of Ukraine's security apparatus, including the head of Ukraine's successor to the KGB, General Ihor Smeshko, in order to discuss the deployment of their services during the forthcoming election campaign. Within three hours, Yushchenko developed a throbbing headache and, on the following day, acute stomach pains. It was not long before his case was diagnosed as severe food poisoning by his Ukrainian doctors.

Yushchenko's symptoms worsened over the next few days. In addition, he soon developed severe back pain and partial paralysis of the left side of his face.

Five days after his dinner meeting, on September 10, Viktor Yushchenko left for Vienna, Austria, to get treatment from the Rudolfinerhaus Klinic. He was examined by a battery of physicians who all agreed that he suffered from acute pancreatitis and interstitial edematous changes (excessive accumulation of fluid in the tissue spaces). His blood was sent to a number of laboratories for further analysis.

He returned to the Ukraine and within a few days started developing a severe rash and epidermal lesions on his face and torso.

By November, the lesions disfigured his face to such an extent that he bore little resemblance to the handsome leader who had attracted such a popular following. He was suffering from severe chloracne—a terrible condition that is a distinctive characteristic of dioxin poisoning. It was the hallmark of the victims of the infamous Seveso industrial dioxin spill.

In that disaster, on July 10, 1976, a high-pressure valve failed at the perfume factory of the Industrie Chimiche Meda Societa Azionaria chemical plant in Meda, Italy, releasing a huge cloud of chemicals containing high levels of dioxin. The toxic cloud was carried southeast by the wind and soon enveloped the town of Seveso and other communities in the area. The cloud eventually contaminated a region with a population of around a hundred thousand, only twelve miles from Milan. No one died as a result of the accident, but 193 victims, most of them children, were severely disfigured by chloracne, an acnelike eruption of blisters, cysts, and pustules associated with overexposure to certain aromatic hydrocarbons, such as dioxins. Today, despite the

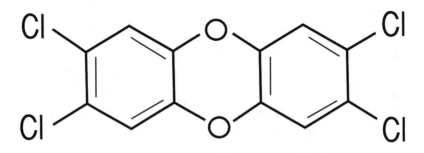

Dioxin, molecular drawing prepared by Morton Satin.

many treatments and operations, the young victims continue to show the ravages of that single exposure to dioxin.

By mid-December 2004, the blood analyses confirmed that Yushchenko's blood contained from six thousand to ten thousand times the normal amount of dioxin. Fortunately, despite his poor health and altered appearance, he returned to the campaign trail. The 2004 Ukrainian presidential election was badly compromised by charges of massive corruption and voter intimidation.

On November 23, 2004, the official results claimed Yanukovych as the winner, but international observers, and all of Yushchenko's supporters, declared the election a fraud. This resulted in a full-blown escalation of the Orange Revolution with widespread protests and civil disobedience. Eventually, the Ukrainian Supreme Court met and annulled the election results and ordered another round of voting for December 26, 2004.

This time, Yushchenko won 52 percent of the vote and was declared the winner on January 10, in the midst of Ukraine's Christmas festivities. Unfortunately, it is impossible to say how long he will continue to suffer the aftereffects of deliberate dioxin poisoning. The victims of the 1976 Seveso disaster continue to suffer disfigurement and other health effects thirty years after the spill.

Yushchenko could easily have died as a result of his September 5 meal with General Smeshko. The general has acknowledged meeting Yushchenko but denies any involvement in the plot to poison him.

As with the case of Georgi Markov, no one knows who wielded the "coward's weapon"—this time placed in food. But, again, as with the case of Markov, we know that the poisoner failed to accomplish the political goals. The Soviet Union collapsed and brought down the Bulgarian government with it. Markov will always be remembered as a hero who tried to gain greater freedom for his fellow citizens. Zhivkov, the Bulgarian Communist Party strongman, has gone down in history as a thug and a dictator. Yushchenko won his election and became his country's leader.

One would think that history has repeatedly demonstrated that the coward's weapon is totally ineffective to accomplish political ends. Killing or attempting to kill individuals ends up as nothing more than an act of personal revenge. Ideas whose time has come are immune to poison. Yet, that doesn't seem to stop the poisoner.

The Alexander Litvinenko Incident

Year	Victim	Poison	Location
2006	Alexander Litvinenko	Polonium-210	London

Alexander V. Litvinenko was born in 1962 in the southwestern Russian city of Voronezh. At the age of eighteen, he graduated from high school and was then drafted into the Internal Troops of the Ministry of Internal Affairs. Five years later, he graduated and became a platoon commander. A year later, in 1986, Litvinenko became an agent for the KGB and was promoted to an operational officer in military counterintelligence.

During the 1990s, Litvinenko moved up the KGB (now FSB) ladder. During that period, he was placed in charge of the protection of Boris Berezovsky, one of perestroika's new multimillionaires, when Berezovsky served the government as secretary of the Security Council. On June 7, 1994, Berezovsky was being driven home in his Mercedes, when his car passed a parked vehicle. A remote-controlled bomb detonated and killed the driver but left Berezovsky untouched. Since the intended victim was of high status, Litvinenko, who by this time had reached the rank of lieutenant colonel, was given the job to investigate the attempted assassination. Thus began the friendship between Litvinenko and Berezovsky.

In 1998 Litvinenko, along with several other officers, accused FSB General Hoholkhov of ordering the assassination attempt on Berezovsky. Despite all the talk of democracy in the new Russia, his pointing a finger at an FSB general was a dangerous act and resulted in the same reaction that it would have during the old KGB days. Litvinenko's testimony marked the immediate end of his career and his new status as a trouble-making dissident.

Like other dissidents in the "new Russia," Litvinenko was continually harassed, intermittently jailed, and forced to sign a document saying he would never defect the country. Boris Berezovsky didn't forget Litvinenko's loyalty and, together with Litvinenko's close friend Alex Goldfarb, arranged for his escape from Russia. In true spy story fashion, Litvinenko fled to Turkey on a false passport and, together with his wife and son, eventually made his way to England, where Berezovsky had settled. There, he asked for political asylum, which was soon granted. It seemed that Litvinenko had really flown over the cuckoo's nest.

In London, Litvinenko renewed his relationship with Berezovsky and other Russian immigrants. He began writing critically of the Russian government and, in particular, of President Vladimir Putin. With the financial support of Berezovsky, Litvinenko published the book *Blowing up Russia: Terror from Within* in 2002, a work extremely critical of the Russian FSB operations against the Chechens.

As time went on, Litvinenko's writing became more shrill and personal. He accused the FSB of being behind the 2002 Chechen Moscow theater hostage drama and the 2005 London subway bombings. He went on to charge that Putin was a pedophile, rapist, and murderer— very strong accusations, even from the relative safety of England.

Just a few weeks before his death, he had begun looking into the shooting death in Moscow of journalist Anna Politkovskaya, who was a fierce and respected critic of Putin and his policies in Chechnya. Friends warned Litvinenko that he had been placed on an FSB hit list.

On November 1, 2006, Litvinenko met at an upscale Mayfair hotel with old FSB colleagues who had come to London to see a soccer match. Afterward, he met Mario Scaramella, an Italian security expert, for lunch at Itsu, a London sushi bar. Later that day, Litvinenko became sick and was admitted to northern London's Barnet General Hospital.

His condition steadily deteriorated and on November 17 he was admitted to University College Hospital in central London. It was clear to physicians that Litvinenko had been poisoned. At first, they thought the poison was thallium, a toxic metal used in rat poisons and insecticides.

Three days later, Litvinenko was moved to intensive care and the press started playing up the story. Representatives of the Russian government said the "theory" that he was poisoned was simply nonsense and contended that he had eaten "bad" sushi.

Two days later, on November 22, Litvinenko's condition deteriorated dramatically. A day later, after wasting away for over three weeks, Alexander Valterovich Litvinenko, forty-three, died of heart failure, leaving behind a wife and a young son.

The diagnosis was no longer thallium poisoning but rather radiation poisoning as a result of ingestion of radioactive polonium-210—which likely originated from a nuclear power plant in Russia. Like radioactive plutonium, polonium-210 is an alpha particle emitter. Alpha particles have low energy, so they cannot penetrate the skin; however, if the particles are inhaled or ingested—as, for example, with food—they can be extremely toxic to the soft, vulnerable internal tissues. It has been estimated that polonium-210 is two hundred and fifty billion times more toxic than hydrogen cyanide.[65]

Polonium was first discovered by Marie and Pierre Curie in 1898. Marie Curie named the radioactive element polonium after her native land of Poland, which was under Russian control at the time. She hoped to highlight her country's lack of independence. What an irony that the very same element was used to kill someone for protesting the excesses and corruption of government in contemporary Russia.

Litvinenko had been administered polonium-210 in some of his food on that fateful November day and suffered the ravages of acute internal radiation poisoning. Once more, the "coward's weapon" was put to use.

As this book goes to press, the investigation into the deliberate radiation poisoning of Alexander Litvinenko widened to include many individuals, countries, and agencies. On Tuesday, May 22, 2007, Britain's Crown Prosecutor charged former KGB officer Andrei Lugovoy with the murder of Litvinenko. Not surprisingly, the Russians refused to allow the extradition of Lugovoy to Britain. We may never know the full circumstances behind the fatal blow to Litvinenko, just as we don't know for certain precisely what happened to Viktor Yushchenko or Georgi Markov. However, we know where the presumption of guilt lies and we also know that the "coward's weapon" will accomplish nothing but immortalization of the victim as a martyr to the concept of democracy and free speech.

When I began writing this book, I never dreamt that my closing paragraphs would be on a political poisoning that had just taken place. Throughout a span of several millennia, food poisoning has been used to attempt to alter the course of history. "Plus ca change, plus c'est la meme chose."

NOTES

1. Fredrick Accum, *A Treatise on Adulterations of Food and Culinary Poisons* (Philadelphia: Abraham Small, 1820).

2. Carl Sandburg, "Always the Young Stranger" *417* (New York: Harcourt Brace, 1952).

3. E. F. Keuchel, "Chemicals and Meat: The Embalmed Beef Scandal of the Spanish-American War," *Bulletin of the History of Medicine* 48, no. 2 (1974): 249–64.

4. H. Zinn, *LaGuardia in Congress*, published for the American Historical Association (Ithaca, NY: Cornell University Press, 1959).

5. H. W. Wiley, *The History of the Crime against the Food Law* (Washington, DC: self-published, 1929).

6. Stuart Chase and F. J. Schlink, *Your Money's Worth; A Study in the Waste of the Consumer's Dollar* (New York: Macmillan, 1927); A. Kallet and F. J. Schlink, *100,000,000 Guinea Pigs* (New York: Grosset & Dunlop, 1933); R. D. Lamb, *American Chamber of Horrors—the Truth about Food and Drugs* (New York: Grosset & Dunlap, 1936).

7. Chase and Schlink, *Your Money's Worth*.

8. Kallet and Schlink, *100,000,000 Guinea Pigs*.

9. Lamb, *American Chamber of Horrors*.

10. C. Ballentine, "Taste of Raspberries, Taste of Death, the 1937 Elixir Sulfanilamide Incident," *FDA Consumer Magazine* (June 1981), http://www.fda.gov/oc/history/elixir.html (accessed August 28, 2006).

11. G. A. Soper, "The Work of a Chronic Typhoid Germ Distributor," *Journal of the American Medical Association* 48 (1907): 2019–22.

12. G. A. Soper, "The Curious Career of Typhoid Mary," *Bulletin of the New York Academy of Medicine* 15 (1939): 698–712.

13. S. J. Baker, *Fighting for Life* (New York: Macmillan, 1939).

14. G. A. Soper, "Typhoid Mary," *Military Surgeon* 45, no. 1 (1919): 1–15.

15. W. H. Park, "Typhoid Bacilli Carriers," *Journal of the American Medical Association* 51 (1908): 982.

16. G. C. Whipple, *Typhoid Fever: Its Causation, Transmission and Prevention* (New York: John Wiley & Sons, 1908).

17. M. L. Ogan, "Immunization in a Typhoid Outbreak in the Sloane Hospital for Women," *New York Medical Journal* 101 (1915): 610–12.

18. G. A. Soper, "The Discovery of Typhoid Mary," *British Medical Journal* 1 (January 7, 1939): 37–38.

19. Baker, *Fighting for Life*.

20. J. P. Morgan, "The Jamaica Ginger Paralysis," *Journal of the American Medical Association* 248, no. 15 (1982): 1864–67.

21. J. P. Morgan and T. C. Tulloss, "The Jake Walk Blues," *Annals of Internal Medicine* 85 (1976): 804–808.

22. Morgan, "The Jamaica Ginger Paralysis."

23. P. M. Wax, "Elixirs, Diluents, and the Passage of the 1938 Federal

Food, Drug and Cosmetic Act," *Annals of Internal Medicine* 122, no. 6 (1995): 456–61.

24. Cyril C. Sullivan, USDA/FDA Chief Inspector, letter to Mr. Haven Parker, Assistant United States Attorney, Boston, MA, March 30, 1932.

25. Ibid.

26. George H. Adams, USDA/FDA Chief, Boston Station, letter to Mr. W. R. M. Wharton, Chief, Eastern District, USDA/FDA, New York, NY, April 7, 1932.

27. J. Parascandola, "The Public Health Service and Jamaica Ginger Paralysis in the 1930s," *PHS Chronicles* 110, no. 3 (1995): 361–63.

28. *Boston Globe*, March 26, 1930; *Boston Herald*, March 27, 1930; *Boston Traveler*, March 27, 1930; *Boston Herald*, March 29, 1930; *Boston Herald*, April 15, 1930.

29. *Boston Herald*, April 14, 1930.

30. Morgan and Tulloss, "The Jake Walk Blues."

31. W. G. Campbell, FDA Chief, Washington, DC, letter to Mr. H. M. Spillers, Secretary of the United Victims of Ginger Paralysis Association, June 9, 1932.

32. W. R. M. Wharton, Chief, Eastern District, USDA/FDA, New York, NY, letter to all stations in the Eastern District, October 28, 1936.

33. Allen Brothers, "Jake Walk Blues," Victor record V-40303, 1930; A. D. Woolf, "Ginger Jake and the Blues: A Tragic Song of Poisoning," *Veterinary and Human Toxicology* 37, no. 3 (1995): 252–54.

34. W. E. Smith and A. Smith, "Death Flow from a Pipe," *Life*, June 2, 1972, pp. 74–79.

35. Out of respect for the family's wishes, I have not placed a copy of the photograph in this book.

36. M. Posada de la Paz, R. M. Philen, and I. A. Borda, "Toxic Oil Syndrome: The Perspective after 20 Years," *Epidemiologic Reviews* 23, no. 2 (2001): 231–27.

37. M. Posada de la Paz et al., "Neurologic Outcomes of Toxic Oil Syndrome Patients 18 Years after the Epidemic," *Environmental Health Perspectives* 111, no. 10 (2003): 1326–34.

38. B. Abaitua et al., "Toxic Oil Syndrome Mortality: The First 13 Years," *International Journal of Epidemiology* 27, no. 6 (1998): 1057–63.

39. B. Wolfenden, "Cover-Up," *Guardian*, August 25, 2001.

40. "Italian Vermouth Tops One Billion Record Exports," Avenue Vine,

http://www.avenuevine.com/archives/000889.html (accessed April 22, 2007).

41. School of International Service, American University, 2006, http://www.american.edu/TED/blowfish.htm (accessed April 24, 2006).

42. Y. Ogura, "Fugu (Puffer Fish) Poisoning and the Pharmacology of Crystalline Tetrodotoxin in Poisoning," in *Neuropoisons*, vol. 1, ed. L. L. Simpson (New York: Plenum Press, 1971), pp. 139–59.

43. C. G. Wood, "The Zombie Poison," *ChemMatters*, American Chemical Society, 2006, Chemistry.Org, http://www.chemistry.org/portal/a/c/s/1/feature_tea.html?id=f216b244f00511d6e2f06ed9fe800100 (accessed April 26, 2006).

44. T. Escherich, "Die Darmbakterien des Neugeborenen und Säuglings," *Fortschritte der Medizin* (Progress in Medicine) 3 (1885): 515–22, 574–54.

45. L. W. Riley et al., "Hemorrhagic Colitis Associated with a Rare Escherichia Coli Serotype," *New England Journal of Medicine* 308, no. 12 (1983): 681–85.

46. "Safeguarding the Food Supply through Irradiation Processing Techniques: An International Conference," Agricultural Research Institute, Orlando, FL, October 25–31, 1992.

47. B. P. Bell et al., "A Multistate Outbreak of Escherichia Coli O157:H7—Associated Bloody Diarrhea and Hemolytic Uremic Syndrome from Hamburgers. The Washington Experience," *Journal of the American Medical Association* 272, no. 17 (1994): 1349–53.

48. T. W. Hennessy et al., "A National Outbreak of Salmonella Enteritidis Infections from Ice Cream. The Investigation Team," *New England Journal of Medicine* 334, no. 20 (May 16, 1996): 1281–86.

49. "Deadly Meat: When a Hamburger Can Kill," transcript 134, *Turning Point*, ABC News, October 20, 1994.

50. Testimony of Diana Nole, *Safe Tables Our Priority (S.T.O.P.)*, http://www.safetables.org/Policy_&_Outreach/Testimony/tt_diana_nole.html (accessed August 26, 2006).

51. Food Safety Initiative Fact Sheet, http://vm.cfsan.fda.gov/~dms/fsfact.html (accessed August 26, 2006).

52. *Federal Register* 63, no. 178 (September 15, 1998): 49359–60.

53. Eddie Collister, "Four Treated for Parasitic Worm as Trail of Student Leads to U.S.," *Globe and Mail* (Toronto), February 27, 1970.

54. Centers for Disease Control and Prevention, http://www.dpd.cdc
.gov/dpdx/HTML/ImageLibrary/Ascariasis_il.asp?body=A-F/Ascariasis
/body_Ascariasis_il11.htm (accessed August 24, 2006).

55. Eddie Collister, "Student Hunted as Would-Be 'Parasite Killer,'"
Gazette (Montreal), February 26, 1970.

56. *Lakeshore News and West Island Chronicle* 18, no. 8, Pointe Claire
(February 26, 1970); *Lakeshore News and West Island Chronicle* 18, no. 9,
Pointe Claire (February 26, 1970).

57. *Lakeshore News and West Island Chronicle* 18, no. 10, Pointe Claire
(February 26, 1970).

58. Leon Levinson, "Kranz Sent to Trial in 'Bug' Murder Try," *Gazette*
(Montreal), March 19, 1970.

59. Lewis F. Carter, *Charisma and Control in Rajneeshpuram* (Cambridge: Cambridge University Press, 1990).

60. Rosemary Hamilton, *Hellbent for Enlightenment: Unmasking Sex,
Power, and Death with a Notorious Master* (Ashland, OR: White Cloud
Press, 1998).

61. Seth Carus, *Bioterrorism and Biocrimes: The Illicit Use of Biological
Agents Since 1900* (Washington, DC: Center for Counterproliferation Research, National Defense University, August 1998–February 2001 Revision).

62. T. J. Torok et al., "A Large Community Outbreak of Salmonellosis
Caused by Intentional Contamination of Restaurant Salad Bars," *Journal of
the American Medical Association* 278, no. 5 (August 6, 1997): 389–95.

63. Frances Fitzgerald, "A Reporter at Large; Rajneeshpuram—I," *New
Yorker*, September 22 and 29, 1986.

64. C. J. S. Thompson, *Poisons and Poisoners* (London: Harold Shaylor,
1931).

65. Anonymous, *New Scientist* (December 2, 2006): 3.

EPILOGUE

Food poisoning, whether unintentional or deliberate, has always had an impact on the course of human events and history. As far back as biblical times, civilized society has been plagued by it. Some of the very same diseases from ancient times exist today, and, strangely enough, the some of our most up-to-date cures could be taken almost verbatim from the Bible.

Certain food and beverage poisonings have had a continual run of two thousand years and throughout that time have not only affected the people of countless societies but have also had an impact on the thinking and behavior of influential leaders. Who knows how different the world would have been had lead poisoning not reduced the intellectual capacities of some of the great Greek and Roman leaders? Empires may have been lost over a few unsuspected molecules.

In every major historical era, foodborne diseases have altered the course of human events. It was not until the last quarter of the nineteenth century that we began to understand the nature of spoilage and disease. Even after we gained this knowledge, we were powerless against the forces of nature exerted through her tiniest beings.

Microorganisms, too small to be seen, have constantly evolved in order to survive. In pursuit of survival, they have developed unique and opportunistic mechanisms that often exceed our technical abilities to control them.

The combination of vast industrialized food production, communal eating in fast-food chains, and terrorists committed to using any means to destroy our lives and lifestyles has resulted in a cocktail of risks such as we have never seen before.

However, a risk is only a risk and not an endpoint. Thus far, we have been reasonably good at or remarkably lucky in avoiding the consequences of these risks. Let us hope we continue to do so.

But we must not take the abundance of safe food and clean water for granted. We must not relax our watchfulness lest we discover that there continues to be Death in the Pot.

INDEX

249